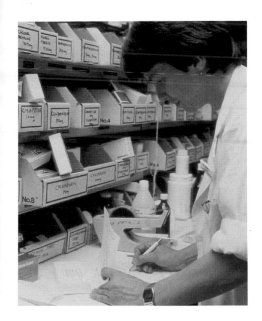

Preface

The Audit Commission has been responsible for the external audit of local authorities in England and Wales since 1983, and in 1990 it assumed responsibility for auditing the NHS. As well as reviewing the financial accounts of local government and health service bodies, the Commission's auditors have a statutory duty to examine the economy, efficiency and effectiveness of the use of resources. The Commission aims to help those who manage and work in local authorities and the NHS to deliver the best possible services with the money that is available so that public expenditure makes the maximum contribution to society.

This report seeks to emphasise to NHS trust boards the importance of medicines management as a very significant part of their clinical governance responsibilities. It is one of a number of complementary initiatives seeking to raise the profile of medicines management:

- in 1999, the Department of Health (DoH) introduced the Controls Assurance Framework, which includes a section devoted to reducing the risk involved in the use of medicines (Ref. 1);

- in 2000/01, hospitals in England have assessed their services against the DoH's Medicines Management Framework, which has highlighted priority action areas (Ref. 2);

- in concert with this exercise, the Audit Commission is currently collecting baseline data about medicines management arrangements, which will enable local auditors to work with hospitals, and with chief pharmacists in particular, to improve services;

- the Audit Commission will work with chief pharmacists' groups to interpret and analyse these data; and

- in 2002, the Audit Commission will produce an internet site to provide guidance on the self-administration of medicines by hospital patients.

This report, and the associated audit guide, data collection and training, was prepared by Michael Yeats, Ian Jones, Amy Kerbel, Emma Cox, and Nick Mapstone with direction from Jonathan Boyce.

A number of individuals have provided support and guidance to the study team as the work has developed. They are listed in Appendix 1, together with the organisations visited and the underlying study methodology. The Commission is very grateful for their contribution though, as always, responsibility for the findings and conclusions of the study rests with the Commission alone.

1

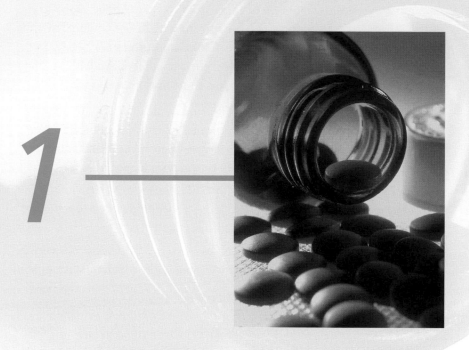

Introduction

Optimising the use of medicines hospitals is central to the
quality of patient care in hospitals. But many hospitals face
significant service pressures that prevent them improving
the quality of care given to patients.

A hospital patient discusses her medication with the healthcare team on their ward round. The pharmacist team-member explains proposed changes to the medication, which the patient will administer herself. The pharmacist also discusses learning points with other team members.

New medication is agreed between members of the clinical team and ordered at the bedside though a radio computer link to an automated dispensary, where robotic systems pick the new medicines and dispatch them to the patient's ward via a pneumatic tube.

Computer technology updates the electronic patient record, to which the patient's GP has access. The medication that has been issued is simultaneously recorded to update stock records and order fresh supplies.

1.   The scenario described above is not necessarily a fanciful vision. The best hospitals in the UK are only a few steps away from working like this. But for many, the vision is a pipe-dream. In these hospitals, many aspects of medicines management arrangements and practice remain rooted in the 1970s. But 30 years ago, the pace of life was slower – the average length of stay in hospital was 15 days and bed occupancy ran at 70 per cent.

2.   Today, average lengths of stay are less than seven days; bed occupancy runs at over 95 per cent in some hospitals; patients are more chronically ill; and are more likely to be transferred between wards. The increased pace and complexity of work means that the use of medicines is not always managed to best effect.

3.   Workload pressures are mounting at a time when medicines are becoming ever-more powerful and complex. This means that the risk of medication errors is increasing, and there are longer delays in supplying medicines. This scenario increases staff stress and turnover, creating a downward spiral that makes significant service improvement a challenge too far.

4.   Great strides are needed to make medicines management practice in all UK hospitals match the level of the best. A definition of medicines management illustrates the extensive and inclusive nature of the agenda [BOX A].

BOX A

Medicines management defined

Medicines management in hospitals encompasses the entire way that medicines are selected, procured, delivered, prescribed, administered and reviewed to optimise the contribution that medicines make to producing informed and desired outcomes of patient care.

Source: Audit Commission

...improved medicines management underpins many of the specific objectives that are set out in the NHS Plan *and* Improving Health in Wales.

5. There are some important obstacles to improving medicines management arrangements:

- many boards are concerned with short-term financial targets and are unwilling or unable to invest money to achieve sustainable quality and cost improvements;

- there are serious recruitment and retention problems in some hospital pharmacy services;

- some pharmacists are content with their traditional dispensing and monitoring functions – the word 'pharmacy' conjures up in their minds a room in a hospital, not a patient-centred service where the pharmacist is a key member of the clinical team; and

- some doctors and nurses have neither the will nor the incentives to change traditional ways of working.

6. But the status quo is unsustainable:

- hospital medication errors are unacceptably common;

- the efficacy of medicines is increasing, but costs are rising;

- the complexity of ensuring the safe use of new medicines is growing; and

- there is an urgent need to review medicines management across whole health economies, as the distinction between primary and secondary care becomes increasingly blurred.

7. Moreover, improved medicines management underpins many of the specific objectives that are set out in the *NHS Plan* and *Improving Health in Wales* (Refs. 3 and 4). For example, these include:

- providing new mechanisms to satisfy patients that the care they get is quality assured;

- reducing the 'postcode lottery' in the prescribing of anti-cancer medicines;

- establishing rapid access to chest-pain clinics;

- ensuring that mental health teams provide an immediate response to crises; and

- reducing the number of patients who are dying or being paralysed from accidents involving spinal injections.

Why has this report been written?

8. This report has important strategic recommendations for the DoH and the National Assembly for Wales (the National Assembly). But it is primarily aimed at board members of NHS trusts, and concentrates on the issues that they have to address. It has two aims:

• to raise the profile of medicines management in hospitals; and

• to make the case for providing adequate investment to enable standards to be raised.

9. All members of the clinical team need to work together to manage medicines effectively. Non-clinical staff too have to ensure effective financial management, procurement and logistics. But before they can succeed, there are systemic and resource issues that boards must address.

10. The strategic challenges facing boards are described, together with the main obstacles and possible solutions. They should use this report to identify how well their hospital manages medicines, what the most important local priorities are, and how to deliver them.

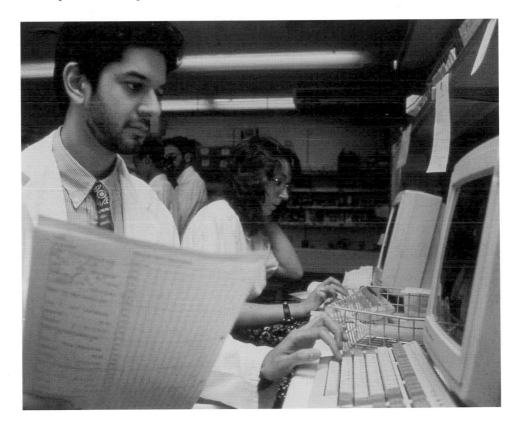

2—

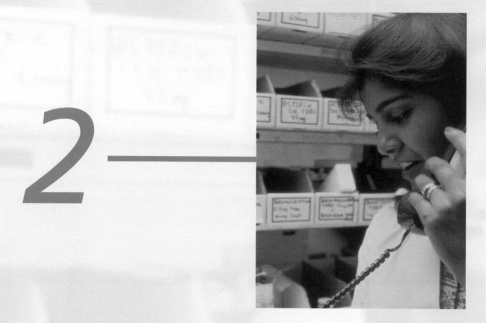

Background

Expenditure on medicines is rising as new therapies are developed and as more patients are being treated. These cost pressures need to be viewed as part of the overall package of patient care – for some conditions, medicines expenditure should be rising because an increase in spending provides a cost-effective way of increasing health gain for the population.

Recent trends

11. Medicines management is central to the quality of healthcare. Nearly all patients are given medication as a result of a visit to hospital – 7,000 individual doses are administered daily in a 'typical' hospital; and up to 40 per cent of nurses' time is spent administering medicines.

12. In 1999/2000, NHS hospitals spent over £1.5 billion on medicines, which accounted for 4.6 per cent of their costs. In addition, pharmacy staff cost £300 million a year.

13. Relative spending on hospital medicines has risen over the last ten years, and in the last five it has outstripped growth in primary care medicines expenditure [**EXHIBIT 1**].

14. Expenditure is rising because:

- new, more expensive therapies are always being developed;
- more patients are being treated;
- the population is ageing and has more chronic illness; and
- medicines are being used in preference to invasive treatments.

EXHIBIT 1

NHS expenditure on medicines by hospitals and its contribution to total NHS medicines expenditure

Spending on medicines rose sharply over the last ten years, and in the last five years it accounted for a steadily increasing percentage of total expenditure on medicines.

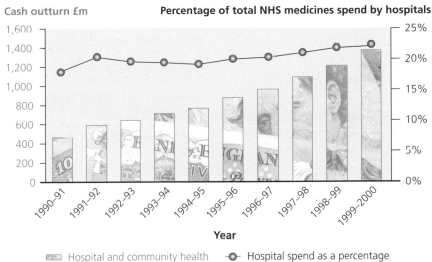

Cash outturn £m — **Percentage of total NHS medicines spend by hospitals**

Year

Hospital and community health services cash outturn — Hospital spend as a percentage of the total

Source: Audit Commission analysis of data obtained from the DoH

For some conditions, medicines expenditure should be rising because it would be a cost-effective way of increasing health gain for the population.

15. There are, of course, differences in the relative amount of money that hospitals spend on medicines. But even after accounting for differences in activity, there remains a significant variation between similar hospitals in the proportion of their non-pay expenditure on medicines [EXHIBIT 2].

16. It is not known how much of the variation is explained by differences in the age and medical condition of the patients treated because:

- hospitals use different descriptions of medicines;
- hospitals do not use a common coding system;
- medicines are commonly used to treat multiple conditions; and
- there are no nationally accepted ways of aggregating data to account for differences in the age or illness of the patients treated.

17. What is clear, however, is that some hospitals are experiencing significant increases in their medicines expenditure [EXHIBIT 3]. In recent years, these cost pressures have been driven by the introduction of new medicines to treat cancer, heart disease, arthritis, and a range of psychiatric conditions. In London alone, expenditure on anti-retroviral medicines for the treatment of AIDS/HIV has risen to £51 million – over one-sixth of the total expenditure on medicines by London hospitals.

18. These cost pressures are cause for concern for many trust boards, but they need to be viewed as part of the overall package of patient care. For some conditions, medicines expenditure should be rising because it would be a cost-effective way of increasing health gain for the population. For example, expenditure on proton pump inhibitors and H2 antagonists should be rising because their use improves the quality of patients' lives and saves money by preventing invasive surgery.

EXHIBIT 2

Proportionate expenditure on medicines

There is a two-fold variation between similar trusts' standardised expenditure on medicines.

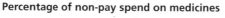

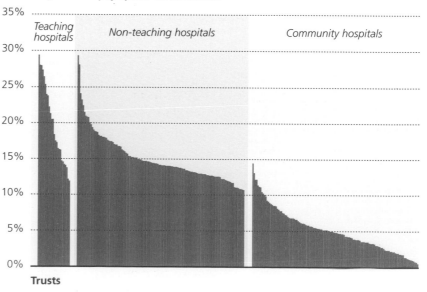

Percentage of non-pay spend on medicines

Teaching hospitals   Non-teaching hospitals   Community hospitals

Trusts

Source: Audit Commission analysis of 1999/2000 TFR3 data

Average increases in medicines expenditure over the last three years

Some trusts have experienced significant increases in medicines expenditure.

Note: N=171

Source: Audit Commission acute hospitals portfolio data

Percentage increase in medicines expenditure 1998/99 to 2000/01

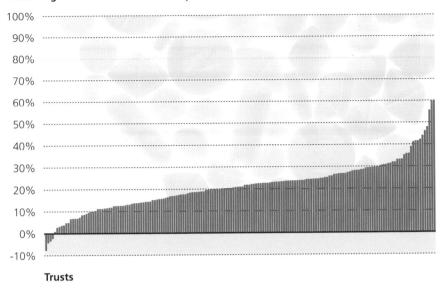

Trusts

Why trust boards should review medicines management arrangements now

19. It is timely for trust boards to review medicines management arrangements because:

- The DoH's report, *An Organisation with a Memory,* found that 10,000 hospital patients each year have serious adverse reactions to medicines, and one-fifth of clinical negligence litigation stems from hospital medication errors (Ref. 5). The Chief Medical Officer has set trusts a target to reduce serious medication errors by 40 per cent by 2005 (Ref. 6).

- Spending on medicines has been identified as a key area for examination by the government's efficiency task force. In response, the DoH has produced a Medicines Management Framework that will be applied to all acute trusts, with reports being made to regional directors of performance review (Ref. 2).

- The report of the *Task and Finish Group for Prescribing in Wales* to the the National Assembly seeks to 'assure high standards in the clinical care of patients and to enhance professional fulfilment in those concerned with patients through the prescribing of medicines' (Ref. 7).

- Medicines management is an important part of the DoH's Controls Assurance Framework, which seeks to manage risk (Ref. 1).

- The recent review of NHS procurement requires all boards to agree a written procurement strategy that includes medicines, as a major expenditure item (Ref. 8).

- New money was announced in the NHS Plan explicitly to improve IT expertise and capacity (Ref. 3). High priority needs to be given to electronic patient records and to electronic prescribing, which should provide significant understanding of the effectiveness of medicines and help to track patients between hospital and primary care.

- The NHS Plan also states that by 2004 over one-half of the nursing workforce, together with pharmacists and allied health professionals, will be able to supply medicines (Ref. 3). This is a major change for which trust boards need to prepare.

- In September 2000, the DoH published *Pharmacy in the Future – Implementing the NHS Plan*, which set out a programme for pharmacy services (Ref. 9). It says that hospital pharmacists will 'ensure that inpatients' medication is got right early in their stay and that they have the medicines they need as soon as they are ready to be discharged.'

- The National Service Framework for Older People emphasises the importance of medicines management arrangements (Ref. 10) **[BOX B]**.

BOX B

National Service Framework for Older People – the relevance of medicines management issues

- As people get older, their use of medication tends to increase. Four in 5 people over 75 take at least 1 prescribed medicine, with 36 per cent taking 4 or more medicines (Ref. 11).

- The ageing process affects the body's capacity to handle medicines.

- Multiple diseases and complicated medication regimes may affect the patients' capacity and ability to manage their own medication regime.

- Adverse reactions are implicated in 5 per cent to 17 per cent of hospital admissions of older people (Refs. 12 and 13).

- While in hospital, 6 per cent to 17 per cent of older inpatients experience adverse drug reactions (Ref. 14).

- As many as 50 per cent of older people do not take their medication as intended (Ref. 15).

- Unintentional changes in medication after discharge from hospital happen too frequently (Ref. 16).

- There is often poor communication between hospital and primary care and vice-versa. Communication needs to be improved to reduce delay in the transfer of medication recommendations to primary care; to ensure treatment that was only intended as short-term, while in hospital, is discontinued on discharge; and to improve explanations of medication changes. In primary care, the interpretation and actioning of discharge medication histories is not always optimal (Ref. 17).

- Older people who are taking four or more medicines have an increased risk of suffering an adverse reaction to a medicine and being readmitted to hospital as a result (Refs. 18 and 19).

- The National Service Framework for Older People states that by 2002, all hospitals should have one-stop dispensing or dispensing for discharge schemes and, where appropriate, self-administration schemes for medicines for older people (Ref. 10).

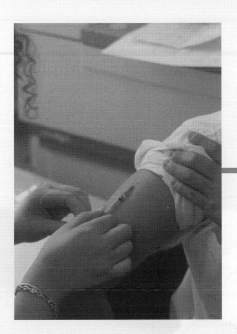

3

Strategic Challenges

Hospitals face several challenges in optimising the use of medicines. They need to link medicines management to clinical governance and, in particular, introduce processes to reduce risk and the number of medication errors. Hospitals must also manage medicines across their local health economies and work with commissioners and primary care to improve financial planning.

20. There are four strategic challenges facing hospitals in relation to medicines:

- linking medicines management to clinical governance;
- managing risk;
- forming effective relationships with primary care; and
- improving financial planning.

Linking medicines management to clinical governance

The role of the trust board in medicines management

21. Under the 1999 Health Act, boards must assure the quality of patient care (Ref. 20). Their clinical governance development plans need to contain specific arrangements to implement quality assurance and monitoring measures for key activities, such as medicines management. These arrangements should supplement and deepen existing professional and statutory controls.

22. Shortcomings in medicines management arrangements are evident in many hospitals:

- Pharmacy services have traditionally established quality control mechanisms, such as prescription monitoring, but these can fall short of the ideal – medicines management now needs to be developed to fit into an overall structure for clinical governance.

- Only 11 out of 105 hospital consultants surveyed in 4 hospitals visited reported that reviews of the use of medicines fed into wider clinical audit work and their clinical governance agendas.

- Reviews of board meetings' minutes show that many have not considered important aspects of medicines management. A common response is that medicines management is the responsibility of Drugs and Therapeutics Committees (DTCs). However, analysis of their activities shows that there are not always systematic reviews of the cost and efficacy of the most significant medicine categories.

- Individual consultants' clinical freedom still takes precedence over corporate clinical responsibility, and prescribing practice is seldom reviewed systematically. Only 9 of 105 consultants surveyed reported that prescribing practice formed part of their regular performance review meetings with clinical directors.

- Information systems have shortcomings: only 17 of 105 consultants surveyed felt that they receive adequate information about how their prescribing practice compares with colleagues in their specialty. Most data that are available relate to the cost of medicines, without proper consideration of their efficacy or health outcomes.

23. These findings suggest that some trust boards are neglecting an important aspect of their clinical governance duties. As a starting point, they should use the DoH's Medicines Management Framework in conjunction with the Audit Commission's diagnostic to monitor medicines management arrangements and develop local action plans **[BOX C]** (Ref. 2).[1]

24. Board-level involvement in medicines management can reduce costs as well as improve quality **[CASE STUDY 1, overleaf]**.

BOX C

Quality standards and targets for medicines management

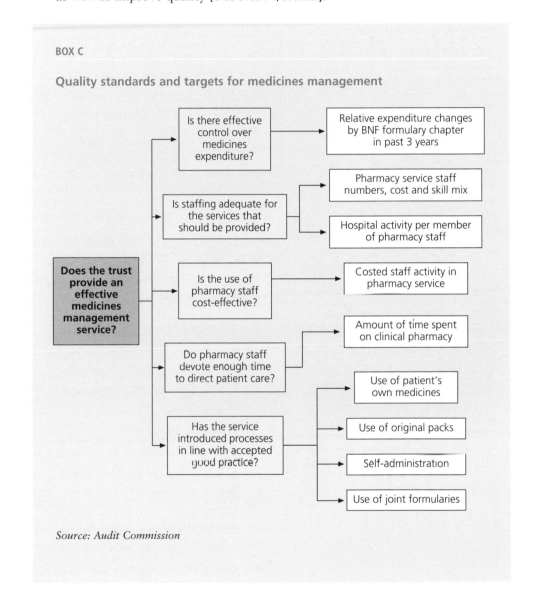

Source: Audit Commission

I   Medicines management is included in the Audit Commission's Acute Hospitals Portfolio – data from all acute trusts on each area referred to in Box C will be collected during 2001. The data will be analysed and the results reported to trusts as part of the 2001/02 audit programme.

North Staffordshire Hospitals NHS Trust – medicines management governance arrangements

To encourage all clinical directorates to focus on prescribing issues, a series of reports are presented quarterly to the board. They include a summary table showing the medicine budgets and actual expenditure for the trust as a whole and for each directorate.

A narrative reporting the recent decisions of the DTC and the Medicines Management Group, as well as identifying key prescribing issues in each directorate, supplements this financial information.

Prescribing is also made a regular feature of performance review meetings between the chief executive and clinical directors.

Better use of medicines has been demonstrated by these actions, and savings have resulted (see Exhibit 11.)

Source: Audit Commission study site

The role of the Drugs and Therapeutics Committee

...establishing an agreed formulary is the cornerstone of effective medicines management.

25. A process of establishing an agreed formulary is the cornerstone of effective medicines management. There are a number of quality and cost consequences if formularies are not developed:

- greater diversity of prescribing practice resulting in an increased risk of medication errors;
- higher medicine costs;
- an increased chance of medicines being out of stock;
- a greater risk of passing medicine expiry dates; and
- higher administrative costs because more lines have to be ordered.

26. An effective DTC will help to ensure that:

- national and locally agreed treatment guidelines are adhered to;
- therapeutic categories with high-risk, high-volume or expensive medicines are regularly reviewed;
- non-formulary medicines are not routinely stocked;
- prescribers are monitored for excessive use of non-formulary medicines;
- the formulary is evaluated periodically for ineffective and obsolete medicines; and
- the quality and cost impact of new medicines is always assessed.

27. In the more progressive hospitals the role of the DTC is developing. A criticism of the traditional formulary is that it is simply a list of medicines: the formulary only becomes a live operational document once the medicines are tied to a diagnosis.

28. Chief executives and medical directors should make the DTC at their trust accountable to the trust board for the introduction of evidence-based formularies which are linked to clinical and National Institute for Clinical Excellence (NICE) guidelines. These should describe how common conditions are to be treated, including the medicines to be used. To ensure the best treatment for patients, the information is best stored in electronic format so that it is available at the time that prescribing decisions are made.

29. These systems will become more important with the growth of prescribing by nurses and other healthcare professionals. The Government has announced that £10 million has been allocated from 2001 to 2004 to train 10,000 nurses (in primary care and in hospitals) to prescribe medicines independently for common conditions in the areas of minor ailments, minor injuries, health promotion and palliative care.

30. DTCs also have a strategic role in monitoring prescribing practice. While detailed analysis is in the domain of clinical audit, the DTC should analyse data on medicines use at an aggregate level, both over time and in comparison to similar hospitals. For example, DTCs might monitor aspects of the hospital's practice with regard to the prescription of antibiotics, an area where there is wide variation between similar trusts [EXHIBIT 4]. Analysis of this sort could generate reviews of local practice.[1]

I High levels of use of antibiotics may not necessarily be 'bad' – it could indicate a successful policy of discharging those patients who can take antibiotics orally.

EXHIBIT 4

Comparison of hospitals' expenditure on antibiotics administered orally vs. intravenously

There is wide variation between similar trusts in the use of oral vs. intravenous antibiotics.

Percentage expenditure on oral vs IV antibiotics

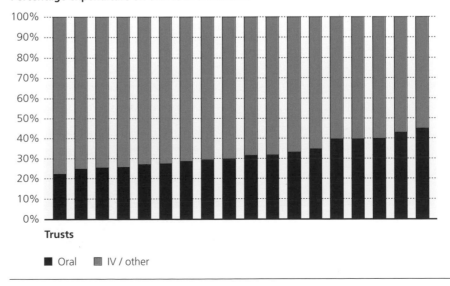

Trusts

■ Oral ■ IV / other

Source: Audit Commission study sites

31. DTCs will increasingly become involved in whole health economy prescribing practice. This development is foreshadowed by the proposal in the Task and Finish Group in Wales that more of DTCs' responsibilities should be devolved to local health groups (LHGs) (Ref. 7).

Risk management

A serious problem?

32. Linking medicines management to clinical governance will help to assure effective clinical practice, and minimise the risk of medication errors,[I] which are an important cause of morbidity in hospitals [BOX D] (Refs. 21, 22, 23, 24). They account for about one-fifth of deaths due to all types of adverse event in hospital and are also an increasingly common stimulus to litigation (Ref. 25).[II]

33. In the USA, the number of deaths because of medication errors and the adverse effects of medicines used in hospitals increased from 2,876 in 1983 to 7,391 in 1993 (Ref. 24). There is also evidence of an upward trend in the UK [EXHIBIT 5]). Such trends may be due to the increasing pace of work in hospitals and to the greater toxicity of modern medicines. During 2001, the DoH has had to publish guidance on preventing medication errors involving spinal injections, in response to a high profile incident (Refs. 28 and 29).

34. Although much of the academic literature on this subject comes from overseas, it is now accepted that these findings can be transferred to the NHS (Ref. 30). It is recognised that medication errors alone cost the NHS about £500 million a year in additional days spent in hospital (Ref. 6).

35. However, the true extent of medication errors is unknown because of inadequate definitions and different reporting arrangements. Only one hospital visited had a comprehensive error and near-miss reporting system in place.

I   A medication error may be defined as '…any preventable event that may cause or lead to inappropriate medication use or patient harm, while the medication is in the control of the health care professional, patient, or consumer. Such events may be related to professional practice, health care products, procedures, and systems including: prescribing; order communication; product labelling, packaging and nomenclature; compounding; dispensing; distribution; administration; education; monitoring; and use'.

II   Medical Defence Union data show that one-quarter of all indemnity paid out following litigation claims after adverse events in general practice results from medication errors. Their contribution to adverse events in hospital is not known but is unlikely to be smaller, in view of the scale and complexity of hospital medicines prescribing. Litigation claims cost the NHS £400 million in 1998/99.

BOX D

Evidence of adverse events in hospitals

From the USA

- Incidence of iatrogenic disease is 4 per cent or 1 million cases per year in the USA[I]
- There are four times as many deaths from iatrogenic disease (180,000 a year) as from road traffic accidents (45,000)
- Over 69 per cent of iatrogenic accidents were considered avoidable
- 20 per cent of adverse events were related to medicines use

Source: Ref. 26

From the UK

- 10.8 per cent of patients on medical wards experience an adverse event, 46 per cent of which were judged to be preventable
- One-third lead to greater morbidity or death
- Each event leads to an average of 8.5 additional days in hospital
- If the data from the sample trusts are representative and extrapolated across the NHS, this costs the NHS £1.1 billion each year
- 12 per cent of adverse events were related to medicines use

Source: Ref. 27

Examples of errors at one hospital

- A patient on the anti-cancer medicine tamoxifen was prescribed the sleeping tablet temazepam instead
- A contraceptive steroid was prescribed instead of an anti-psychotic injection
- A toxic medicine to be given weekly was prescribed daily
- An anti-cancer medicine was prescribed at 1,000 times the correct dose

Source: Clinical audit review at one study site

I   Iatrogenic disease is that caused by a clinician's intervention.

EXHIBIT 5

The number of deaths in England and Wales from medication errors and the adverse effects of medicines, 1990 to 2000

The number of reported deaths shows an upward trend.

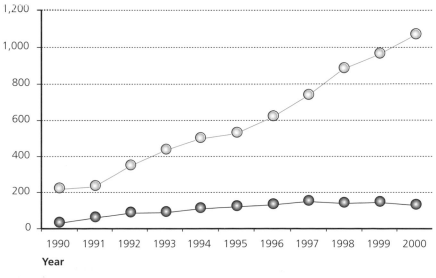

Number of deaths

Source: ICD9 and ICD10 data

36. The DoH's proposals to address these issues centre upon the establishment of the National Patient Safety Agency. The establishment of standard nation-wide definitions and categories of medication errors and 'near-misses' should be an early priority for the Agency. Trusts should be required to adopt such systems as part of their clinical governance arrangements and report progress in their annual reports, as well as reporting along the lines proposed in *Building a Safer NHS* (Ref. 6).

37. Following agreement of standard definitions and categories of medication errors, baseline audits should be undertaken with central funding at a representative sample of hospitals. This will calibrate the current situation in order that improvement targets can be set and their achievement monitored. Work should prioritise specialties or areas with the highest likely risk (for example, ITUs, paediatrics, antibiotics, and nutrition).

The pharmacist's role in reducing medication errors

38. Pharmacists have traditionally had an important quality control role in checking patients' medication. Typically, between one-fifth and one-quarter of inpatient prescription charts are amended by pharmacists for a variety of reasons that reflect shortcomings in the basic rules for safe prescribing [EXHIBIT 6].

EXHIBIT 6

Nature of errors on medicine charts identified by pharmacists

Prescription charts are amended by pharmacists for a variety of reasons.

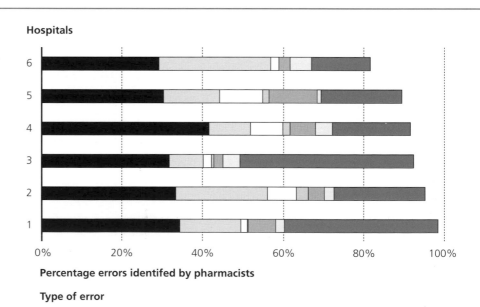

Hospitals

Percentage errors identifed by pharmacists

Type of error

- ■ Patient's name incorrect
- ☐ Dose incorrect
- ☐ Frequency of dose incorrect
- ☐ Administration route incorrect
- ▨ Form of drug incorrect
- ☐ Adverse drug reaction warning
- ▨ Other errors

Source: Analysis of data collected from six hospitals in the Oxford region

39. Concerns have recently been expressed that the core curricula at medical schools do not provide a thorough knowledge of safe medicines prescribing and administration (Ref. 31). Shortcomings in doctors' knowledge means that there is a particular risk of medication errors when they first arrive in hospital. Only a small proportion of new doctors believe that their induction dealt adequately with medicines management issues [EXHIBIT 7].

40. Medication errors are common because of major systemic weaknesses in prescribing arrangements. About 70 per cent of prescribing decisions are made by house officers and senior house officers even though they have little experience of medicines. Studies have also shown that they are prone to increasing error rates when they are stressed, tired, distracted, or are working in unfamiliar surroundings – almost a stereotype of hospital life (Refs. 32 and 33).

Can medication errors be avoided?

41. It is important not to under-estimate the task of minimising medication errors. The prescriber has to be knowledgeable enough to choose an effective treatment that is suitable for the individual patient, taking into account age, infirmity, and possible interactions with other medicines. Having selected the right medicine and the correct dose, the prescriber has to transmit the message to the dispenser. They then have to hand the medicine to the patient, or to a carer or nurse, who has to see that the medicine is given in the correct way and at the specified times.

EXHIBIT 7

The perceptions of doctors in training of support in medicines management issues

Only a small proportion of doctors in training report that their induction dealt adequately with medicines management issues.

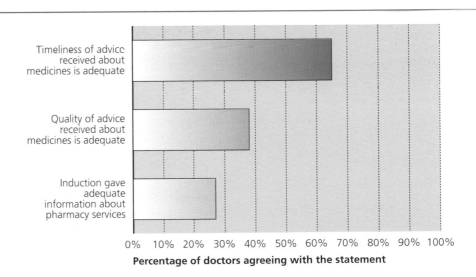

Percentage of doctors agreeing with the statement

Source: Audit Commission study sites

...senior managers should also seek assurance that actual clinical practice reflects agreed protocols.

42. Medication errors occur because of the complexity of this process, but there are several ways in which risk can be minimised:

- changing the risk management culture;

- induction and training;

- redesigning processes and using computer technology to reduce errors; and

- developing clinical pharmacy services.

Changing the risk management culture

43. A typical response to errors in hospitals is to identify those involved and castigate them (Ref. 26). The UKCC has recorded its concern that nurses who made mistakes under pressure of work, and were honest and open about those mistakes to senior staff, have often been subject to disciplinary action. This discourages incident reporting and is potentially detrimental to patient care.

44. Hospitals need to learn from the practices of other high-risk industries where risk management concentrates on 'near misses' as a way of reducing systemic errors (Ref. 34). The government's view of clinical governance emphasises the need to adopt *'a systematic approach to quality assurance and improvement ... above all, clinical governance is about changing organisational culture ... away from a culture of blame to one of learning so that quality infuses all aspects of the organisation's work'*(Ref. 3).

45. Trust boards should distinguish between cases where the error is the result of reckless practice and those that have been the result of serious pressure of work and where an immediate, honest disclosure is made. All errors and incidents require thorough and careful investigation that takes full account of the circumstances and context of the event and the underlying systemic causes.

46. Trust boards and senior managers should also seek assurance that actual clinical practice reflects agreed protocols. The recent events at Queen's Medical Centre illustrate how day-to-day pressures can lead to acknowledged best practice being ignored (Ref. 35). There were particular concerns expressed at some hospitals visited of aseptic preparations being made-up on wards, despite protocols stating that they would be prepared in the safer, better quality-assured, facilities in pharmacies. Such practice has been shown to represent a significant risk to patients because of the risks of microbial and medication errors associated with the preparation of intravenous medicines at ward level (Ref. 36).

Induction and training

47. Lead clinicians must ensure that all new clinical staff are provided with a formal induction, which should include the provision of guidelines and protocols covering prescribing practice, medicines administration and error reporting arrangements. New members of staff should sign to acknowledge receipt and understanding of the guidelines. Induction courses should also introduce new clinicians to contact points in the hospital's pharmacy service.

48. After initial induction, there is a need for continuing training and competency assessments for all clinicians who are involved in the prescription and administration of medicines. No one can prespecify their own ignorance, so constant vigilance and a robust safety culture will always be required to prevent accidents.

Redesigning processes and using computer technology to reduce errors

49. Complications arising from medicines treatment are the most common cause of adverse events in hospital patients (Refs. 37 and 38) and generate adverse publicity for the NHS [BOX E]. Errors may occur from the initial decision to prescribe to the final administration of the medicine, and these include choice of the wrong medicine, dose, route, form, and frequency or time of administration (Refs. 39 and 40).

50. Most errors are caused by the prescriber not having immediate access to accurate information about either the medicine (its indications, contraindications,[1] interactions, therapeutic dose, or side effects); or the patient (allergies, other medical conditions, or the latest laboratory results) (Refs. 40, 41 and 42).

---

1   Contraindication – any condition that renders a particular line of treatment improper or undesirable.

BOX E

Examples of adverse publicity involving medication errors

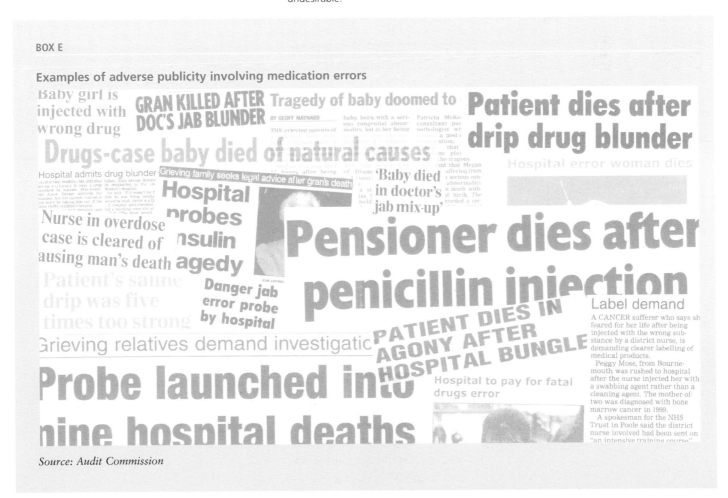

Source: Audit Commission

51. Hand-written prescriptions or patients' notes also contribute to errors as they may be illegible, incomplete, subject to transcription errors or make use of inappropriate 'shorthand' [BOX F]. Prescription sheets themselves may also be temporarily unavailable or lost. To add to the risk of confusion, different medicines are sometimes contained in similar packages [BOX G].

BOX F

Example of patient's notes

Hand-written prescriptions or patients' notes also contribute to errors as they may be illegible, incomplete, subject to transcription errors or may make use of inappropriate 'shorthand'.

Source: Audit Commission study site

BOX G

Example of different medicines in similar packaging

Different medicines are sometimes contained in similar packages.

The packaging of these medicines is almost the same, but prochlorperazine is an anti-emetic medicine to treat nausea or vertigo; and procyclidine is a medicine for treating Parkinson's disease.

Prochlorperazine Tablets BP
5mg
Each tablet contains Prochlorperazine Maleate BP 5mg
They also contain lactose

28 tablets in blister packs

Please read the enclosed leaflet before you start to take this medicine

PATIENT PACK
NORTON X

Procyclidine Tablets BP
5mg
Each tablet contains Procyclidine Hydrochloride BP 5mg
They also contain lactose, microcrystalline cellulose

28 tablets in blister packs

Please read the enclosed leaflet before you start to take this medicine

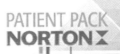

PATIENT PACK
NORTON X

Source: Audit Commission study site

52. Electronic prescribing reduces medicine errors significantly by providing timely, legible information (Refs. 43 and 44). One study concluded that improved information systems could contribute to the prevention of 78 per cent of transcription errors leading to adverse medicine events (Ref. 40). Computerised systems containing rules to prevent incorrect or inappropriate prescribing have also reduced the incidence of errors and increased the appropriateness of medicine treatment (Refs. 45, 46, 47, 48, 49, 50 and 51).

The role of clinical pharmacy in reducing risk

53. Clinical pharmacy applies pharmaceutical expertise to help to maximise medicine efficacy and minimise medicines toxicity in individual patients. It allows pharmacists to become part of the clinical team and to anticipate medication errors. One of the pharmacist's traditional roles is one of quality control, monitoring and reporting on errors only retrospectively. Clinical pharmacy is a move away from re-active quality control towards pro-active involvement in direct patient care and the anticipation of errors.

54. DoH policy has long recognised the importance of clinical pharmacy in minimising both clinical and financial risk (Ref. 52). Enabling pharmacists to contribute more fully to patient care reduces patient morbidity and saves money [**BOX H**] (Ref. 53). In particular, the presence of a pharmacist on ward rounds as a full member of the patient care team reduces prescribing errors significantly (Ref. 54). However, there is wide variation in the amount of time that hospital pharmacists devote to clinical pharmacy [**EXHIBIT 8**].

BOX H

Analysis of clinical pharmacy services that reduce mortality

Clinical pharmacy service	Number of hospitals	Significance[I]	Lives saved[II]
Clinical research	108	P<0.0001	21,125
Medicines information services	237	P<0.043	10,463
CPR team	282	P<0.039	5,047
Medicines history taken on admission	30	P<0.005	3,843

Source: Ref. 53

[I] The 'p' values refer to associations between a particular pharmacy service being present and adjusted mortality rates – there is not necessarily a causal link.

[II] Calculated from the difference in death rate/admission (presence or absence of the clinical service) * mean number of admissions/hospital/year offering the clinical service.

EXHIBIT 8

Proportion of time spent on clinical pharmacy activities

There is wide variation in the proportion of time that pharmacists devote to clinical pharmacy.

Note: N=183

Source: Audit Commission acute hospitals portfolio data

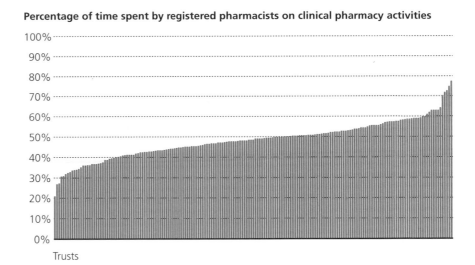

Percentage of time spent by registered pharmacists on clinical pharmacy activities

Trusts

55. Clinical pharmacy activities should also be extended to pharmacist prescribing and to taking patients' medication histories. There is evidence that pharmacists are five times more accurate than doctors in writing discharge prescriptions (Ref. 55). Where it is properly planned and supported, investment in clinical pharmacy improves the quality of patient care and reduces costs **[CASE STUDY 2] [EXHIBIT 9, overleaf)** (Ref. 56).

CASE STUDY 2

North Staffordshire Hospitals NHS Trust – The impact of clinical pharmacy

The medical directorate of the trust, which spends over £1 million annually on medicines, decided to purchase additional pharmaceutical support to provide an experienced clinical pharmacy service to all its wards.

Two senior pharmacists were recruited, with the expectation that they would save more than the cost of their salary each year.

The initiative has reduced prescribing costs by around 25 per cent through more appropriate prescribing.

The greatest savings came from appropriate reductions in poly-pharmacy where patients had been given cocktails of medicines that were designed to overcome the problems caused by other medicines.

Source: Audit Commission study site

EXHIBIT 9

The impact of the introduction of clinical pharmacy

The initiative has reduced prescribing costs by around 25 per cent.

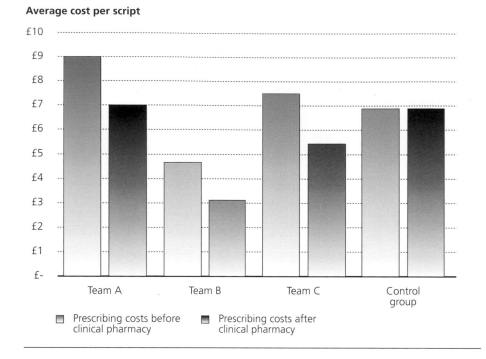

Average cost per script

Source: North Staffordshire Hospitals NHS Trust (Ref. 57).

56. Trusts should undertake reviews of pharmacy staffing levels and consider whether there are adequate resources to:

*   provide all aspects of clinical pharmacy services;

*   meet the demands on pharmacy services of the NHS Plan in respect of new consultants and nurse prescribers (Ref. 3);

*   take patients' medication histories; and

*   support dispensing for discharge schemes.

Forming effective relationships with primary care

57. The third strategic challenge facing trusts is to build effective relationships with primary care in order to improve quality and reduce costs across the local health economy. This requires appropriate **joint-working arrangements** between primary and secondary care and progress in four key inter-related areas:

*   Patients' own medicines

*   Medication review on admission

*   Self-administration

*   Original pack dispensing

Joint-working arrangements

58. Since 1st April 1999, healthcare allocations have been unified across hospital, community health services and general medical services. This means that prescribing costs across health economies are now ultimately cash-limited. Hospitals now have a vested interest in helping to manage GPs' expenditure on medicines.

...some health authorities have appointed medicines management liaison pharmacists to establish more effective joint working...

59. In the past, there were incentives for hospitals to serve their own limited interests, rather than the NHS as a whole, by passing on the cost of medicines to primary care. Suppliers traditionally discounted the price of medicines to hospitals in anticipation of recouping their margins from primary care.

60. GP prescribing is greatly influenced by events and decisions taken in hospitals. About 18 per cent of GP prescribing is hospital-initiated; and 40 per cent is strongly influenced by hospitals, since a GP's choices of medicines is likely to be guided by local consultants' treatment protocols (Ref. 58). Many medicines that are prescribed by hospital doctors are continued for some years after discharge. However, three out of four GPs surveyed said that their local hospital did not take account of the impact on primary care when new medicines were introduced.

61. To tackle these shortcomings, some health authorities have appointed medicines management liaison pharmacists to establish more effective joint working between hospitals and primary care groups or trusts (PCG/Ts); or LHGs in Wales. DTCs also have an important liaison role, and should include representatives from commissioners, GPs, PCGs and community pharmacists to co-ordinate policy. Joint-care protocols should be established to manage formularies and the choice of medicines. These need to develop rapidly through the intermediate stage of disease management guidelines to the eventual objectives of integrated care pathways.

62. 'Whole system prescribing' arrangements should be examined by all health economies, as there is evidence that this approach improves prescribing and saves money [**CASE STUDY 3**].

CASE STUDY 3

Northamptonshire Prescribing Project Group

The Northamptonshire Prescribing Project Group was established at the end of 1999 to advise on prescribing initiatives across the county. The Group comprises representatives from hospitals, PCTs and the health authority.

The Group's work has focused on such issues as therapeutic switching of medicines, introducing branded generic medicines, introducing original pack dispensing and improved information about medicines when patients are discharged from hospital.

The Group has concentrated on agreeing prescribing policies across primary and hospital care, to avoid unnecessary therapeutic 'switching' of medicines when patients move between sectors.

This work has identified bankable savings of £500,000 (from a total medicines expenditure of £60.3 million) by agreeing protocols on the use of medicines for eight conditions in the last 18 months.

Source: Audit Commission study site

63. Despite such clear benefits, progress with introducing such joint arrangements is patchy, as is shown by the development of joint formularies [EXHIBIT 10].

64. Whole system reviews of medicines management practice will also raise fundamental questions about who does what. In particular, the practice of outpatient dispensing by hospitals should be questioned, and indeed has been challenged by the *Report of the Task and Finish Group for Prescribing in Wales* (Ref. 7).

65. There is a logic that says hospitals should dispense only to those outpatients in immediate need, or where the medication is particularly specialised. All other outpatients are their GP's responsibility, with whom the prescribing decision should reside, with advice following the outpatient consultation. Such arrangements would eliminate much of the confusion that is commonly generated when two doctors are prescribing to the same patient.

Patients' own medicines

66. Trusts usually ask patients to take all their medicines into hospital with them so that an accurate medication record can be made. Patients take some £90 million worth of GP-prescribed medicines with them into hospital each year – many of these medicines are destroyed or are not returned when the patient is discharged (Refs. 58, 59 and 60).

67. If patients' medicines are checked on admission by someone who is properly trained, their suitability for reissue can be assessed and such waste can be prevented. Medication should be only designated unsuitable for re-use if:

- there is insufficient quantity;
- the dosage is changed;

EXHIBIT 10

The introduction of joint formularies

The introduction of joint formularies is patchy.

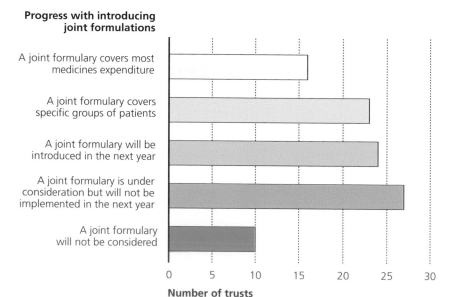

Progress with introducing joint formulations

	Number of trusts
A joint formulary covers most medicines expenditure	16
A joint formulary covers specific groups of patients	23
A joint formulary will be introduced in the next year	24
A joint formulary is under consideration but will not be implemented in the next year	27
A joint formulary will not be considered	10

Note: N=183

Source: Audit Commission acute hospitals portfolio data

- medicine is stopped;
- use-by dates have expired;
- tablets in the container are mixed;
- there is evidence of physical deterioration;
- the medicine is inadequately labelled; or
- the container had no label or batch number.

68. Observing these basic rules offers a significant quality improvement and requires an early assessment of each patient by a pharmacist. They also empower patients and reduce the confusion and errors that can occur when patients receive the same medicines presented and packed in three or four different ways over the space of a few weeks.

69. Re-use of patients' own medicines may save money. One study found that 77 per cent of patients' own medicines were suitable for re-use on admission; and on receipt of the discharge prescription, 56 per cent were re-issued (the balance was not re-issued mainly because the medication was stopped) (Ref. 65). An annual saving of £46,000 was achieved. Another study found that 58 per cent of patients brought some of their medicines into hospital with them, of which 60 per cent were suitable for re-use, yielding the potential to save £37,000 a year in one trust.

Medication review on admission

...30 per cent of patients had incorrect or incomplete medicines or allergies recorded on admission.

70. The National Service Framework (NSF) for Older People requires that hospitals put in place systems for medication review on admission to identify medicines-related problems. This is an area where pharmacists have a vital role, either as provider or trainer. At some hospitals visited, 30 per cent of patients had incorrect or incomplete medicines or allergies recorded on admission. This can lead to poorer quality of care, and longer stays in hospital.

71. Medication review on admission by a pharmacist can also identify whether an admission is due to prescribing errors or to adverse reactions to medicines in the community. Medication review on admission can help to identify such problems and report them back to GPs.

72. The public needs to be made aware of the importance of taking *all* medication (including complementary therapies) into hospital so that patients' own medicines can be used and accurate medicine histories taken. National co-ordination of publicity posters to support an awareness campaign would be worthwhile.

Self-administration of medicines

Patients should not be the passive recipients of prescribing decisions by doctors...

73. The conventional method of giving medicines to patients in hospital is characterised by the use of lumbering drug trolleys on the medicines round. However, the increasing number and complexity of medicines means that this system can no longer support safe or efficient medicines administration.

74. A central theme of both the *NHS Plan* and *Improving Health in Wales* is empowering patients to take an active role in managing their own care (Refs. 3 and 4). Patients should not be the passive recipients of prescribing decisions by doctors – a shared approach needs to be encouraged whereby patients can learn about and take responsibility for their own medication (Ref. 62).

75. Self-administration in hospital allows patients greater independence and enables them to participate in their own care and make decisions about their treatment in partnership with clinical staff. Over 80 per cent of the 350 GPs surveyed supported the introduction of self-administration of medicines by patients in hospital.

76. Self-administration improves patient compliance with medication regimes and so prevents treatment failure (Refs. 63, 64 and 65). In a study of patients with renal failure, 18 per cent did not comply with their medication: 96 per cent of those who did not take their medication as recommended died or had their transplant rejected, compared with 18 per cent of the patients who did (Ref. 66). Another study found that only one-half of patients took their medication properly once they had left hospital (Ref. 67). The failure of patients and clinicians to reach concordance about medication regimes is a major cause of increased morbidity and cost.

77. Almost all patients who self-administer prefer it because it gives them more control. In one study, over 40 per cent of patients felt more confident about taking their medicines when at home, and the same number thought that it had increased their understanding – 90 per cent of self-administering patients knew the purpose of their medicines compared with 46 per cent in a control group (Ref. 68).

78. Self-administration is also beneficial to patients because it:

- enables the medication to do its job – patients can take analgesics when they are in pain, sedation when they want to sleep, and tablets that need to be taken before, with or after food, at the correct time;

- simplifies the medicines regime – many patients, especially older patients, have a number of different diseases all requiring different medicines. The resulting *polypharmacy* leads to patients taking many medicines of doubtful value (Ref. 69). Self-administration leads to simpler and better medicine regimes because fuller assessment of all the patient's medication is required (Ref. 70). Simplification improves compliance with the medication regimen – the rate of non-compliance rises from 15 per cent when patients are asked to take one medicine, to 35 per cent if more than five medicines are prescribed (Ref. 71);

- allows patients to practise taking medicine under supervision – including opening containers, a serious obstacle for some older patients; and

- alerts healthcare staff to any problems the patient may experience with medication.

79. Improved compliance has quality and cost benefits, particularly by preventing readmission – one-quarter of hospital readmissions are because of non-compliance with medicines regimes (Ref. 72). However, progress with implementing self-administration is variable, and there is scope to adopt more progressive policies in some trusts [EXHIBIT 11].

80. The main problem associated with introducing self-administration is the initial investment in time and money that is required. Each patient must have his or her own lockable bedside cupboard at a cost of about £30 each. In view of the likely significant demand for these lockers from hospitals, the NHS Purchasing and Supply Agency should consider establishing a national contract.

81. Investment in staff time is also needed. In hospitals where it has been successfully established, the change process was supported by at least one senior nurse and one clinical pharmacist was solely allocated to the task. Once established, self-administration in an average-sized hospital needs to maintain most of this resource to train new staff, audit performance and ensure that there is continuous improvement.

82. Where such investment is not forthcoming, self-administration schemes invariably fail. Typically, they are left in limbo with the policy practised on some wards, some of the time – a recipe for confusion and increased risk to patients.

EXHIBIT 11

Self-administration of medicines by patients in hospital

Progress with implementing self-administration is variable.

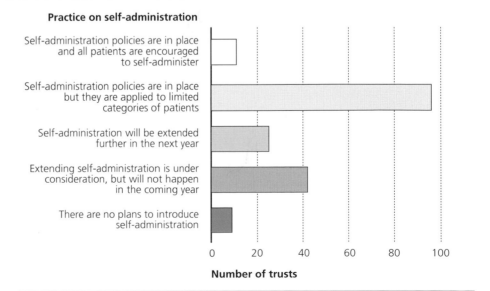

Practice on self-administration

Number of trusts

Note: N=183

Source: Audit Commission acute hospitals portfolio data

Original pack dispensing

83. Closer co-operation across healthcare sectors will promote prescribing and dispensing practice that minimises the cost to the NHS as a whole. In the last ten years, there has been considerable debate about the quantities of medicines issued to patients when they are discharged. DoH guidance was that hospitals should provide a minimum of one week's worth of medicines to patients on discharge (and two weeks' for outpatients) (Ref. 73). But many regions drew up their own detailed guidelines, and some hospitals reduced the quantity of medicines they dispensed in order to cut costs.

84. Such practice served only to increase overall prescribing costs as hospitals are able to buy some medicines at a substantial discount. It was also inconvenient for patients and put an added burden on primary care as each patient had to visit their GP for a repeat prescription, and then obtain the medicine from a community pharmacist.

85. Co-operation between primary and secondary care is imperative because of European Community Directive 92/27, which was incorporated into UK law on 1st January 1999. It requires, among other things, that all medicines supplied to patients include a patient information leaflet (PIL) in appropriate lay language; and be labelled with the product's batch number and expiry date.[I] The Directive is one of the key drivers behind the introduction of original pack dispensing, as the packs contain the leaflets and the expiry date. Most manufacturers supply tablets and capsules in blister-packs for 28 days' treatment, not in bulk.

86. Where trusts' current arrangements limit discharge or outpatient dispensing to one or two weeks' supply, they will have to split some packs and risk non-compliance with the law and possible prosecution. Increasing the dispensed quantity to allow original packs to be used is the only practical solution.

Dispensing medicines to patients in original packs has important benefits...

87. Dispensing medicines to patients in original packs (combined with storing medication at the patient's bedside) has some important benefits, and is in compliance with EU regulations:

- reduced process costs as medicines are dispensed only once;
- greater convenience for patients;
- reduced GP workload at discharge;
- reduced overall costs of medicines to the local health economy because hospital prices are usually lower than those available to GPs;
- having been issued with 28 days' supply on admission, most patients will have left at least two (and on average three) weeks' supply when they are discharged, so allowing time for GPs to be fully informed of any problems or changes in treatment before the patient presents for a repeat prescription;
- reductions in medicine administration error rates (from 9.7 per cent to 2.5 per cent at one study site);

I   There is an exemption for hospital inpatients in that whilst the information needs to be available, the PIL does not need to be physically supplied to each patient.

- hospital discharge is less likely to be delayed as medicines are readily available at the patient's bedside;

- the opportunity for greater use of patients' own medicines as the new system is implemented; and

- fewer interruptions to medical rounds while nurses find medicines from ward stocks.

88. The savings to individual health economies from introducing original pack dispensing will vary. However, work undertaken at one 1,500-bed trust estimated an overall saving of £200,000 a year to the local health economy through better procurement. Trusts will need to discuss local implementation with their health authorities and PCG/Ts, particularly the transfer of money from primary care to hospitals and the consequent impact on GP budgets.

89. Patients are missing the quality improvement that can be derived from original pack dispensing because some health authorities, PCTs/LHGs and hospitals are unable to agree the reallocation of money. Currently, trusts are not maximising their use of original packs [EXHIBIT 12].

90. Original pack dispensing means that hospitals take on more responsibility for dispensing medicines that will be taken in the community. This, in turn, is leading some manufacturers to review their long-standing practice of discounting the cost of medicines to hospitals (in anticipation of recouping their profits from community sales). The resultant reduction in price differentiation between the hospital and the community sector highlights the existing anomaly that hospitals have to pay VAT on the medicines they buy, while the community sector does not. The DoH and the National Assembly need to work with HM Customs and Excise to equalise tax treatments between the sectors and remove what is becoming an obstacle to best prescribing practice.

EXHIBIT 12

The proportion of trusts' total expenditure on medication supplied to patients in original packs

Not all trusts are maximising their use of original packs.

Note: N=182

Source: Audit Commission acute hospitals portfolio data

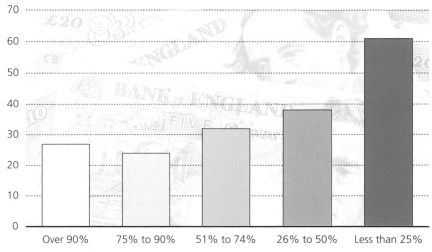

Number of trusts

Percentage of total medicines expenditure spent on medicines in original packs

(categories: Over 90%, 75% to 90%, 51% to 74%, 26% to 50%, Less than 25%)

Integrating initiatives

91. The important point about the innovations described above is that they complement each other. Progress is best achieved, therefore, when they are introduced as part of an integrated strategy [EXHIBIT 13] and [CASE STUDY 4].

EXHIBIT 13

Integrating initiatives in order to deliver better healthcare for patients

Initiatives need to be integrated to deliver the greatest benefit.

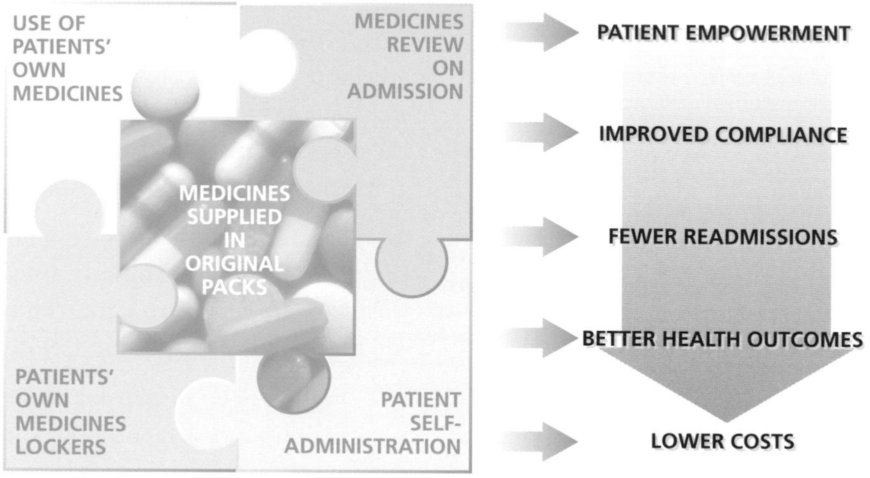

USE OF PATIENTS' OWN MEDICINES

MEDICINES REVIEW ON ADMISSION

MEDICINES SUPPLIED IN ORIGINAL PACKS

PATIENTS' OWN MEDICINES LOCKERS

PATIENT SELF-ADMINISTRATION

PATIENT EMPOWERMENT

IMPROVED COMPLIANCE

FEWER READMISSIONS

BETTER HEALTH OUTCOMES

LOWER COSTS

Source: Audit Commission

CASE STUDY 4

Redesign of medicines supply services at Mid-Sussex NHS Trust

Medicines supply processes have been re-engineered to enhance the role of pharmacy technicians so that time is released for registered pharmacists to spend on clinical pharmacy and direct patient care. The initiative sought to tackle several problems:

- prescribing errors were being made when patients were admitted to hospital because of inadequate information (one-quarter of planned patient admissions did not have accurate information from GPs about their current medication);

- medication and patient selection errors during medicines rounds accounted for over one-quarter of reported medication errors;

- GPs complained about the poor quality of discharge summaries;

- one quarter of re-admissions of elderly care patients were known to be due to failures surrounding medication due partly to lack of information sent to GPs on changes in medication during inpatient stays. An audit at Mid-Sussex found that 31 per cent of emergency medical admissions, whose medicines were changed in hospital, reverted to pre-admission therapy within two weeks of discharge when the GP repeat prescribing system was used to continue treatment;

- waste of inpatient medicines – if a patient moved wards, new medicines were supplied and original medicines destroyed;

...costs were offset by a £60,000 saving from using patients' own medicines...

- a 50 per cent increase in dispensary workload between 1993 and 1998; and

- little control over the timing of dispensary workload.

The trust's aim was to tackle all these problems as part of a 'whole-system' approach, not on a piecemeal basis. All the initiatives taken were based upon existing good practice elsewhere.

The solution

i)   Better use of the skills available

The role of pharmacy technicians has been developed to enable them to assume control of the medicines supply function, thereby releasing registered pharmacists' time to develop their role in:

- reducing patient risk through active involvement in decision making about medicines use; and

- identifying and correcting weaknesses in medicines use by improving prescription monitoring and clinical audits.

A senior technician was made responsible for all operational aspects of the dispensary. A registered pharmacist is available, but her role is primarily to:

- validate any prescriptions that arrive in the dispensary that have not previously been validated by a ward-based pharmacist;

- deal with clinical issues surrounding prescriptions; and

- train and mentor technicians in patient counselling.

ii) Re-engineering the ward-based supply process

Supply processes were changed to:

- use patients' own medication during inpatient stays as the 'lever' for initiating change;

- refocus technicians' work on assessing the suitability for use of patients' own medication for use;

- provide individual de-mountable bedside patient medicines cabinets which 'followed the patient' during their inpatient stay;

- supply medicines ready labelled for discharge to cover both inpatient and immediate post-discharge periods; and

- give GPs and community pharmacists detailed medicines information for patients who had new medication, or who had stopped or changed medicines during their inpatient stay.

There was an increase in costs associated with the initiative: an extra technician was recruited, some existing staff were regraded, and patient lockers were installed. However, these costs were offset by a £60,000 saving from using patients' own medicines, which now account for 10 per cent of items used in the trust. Technicians are now allied with ward-based pharmacists and visit wards on scheduled visits to record details of patients' medication, identifying medication that had been brought in by the patient and medicines that the trust must supply.

contl.

The technician's record is used to supply the medicines to cover the inpatient stay and the immediate period after discharge. These arrangements:

- enable more control of dispensary workflow and remove periods of excessive activity; and

- mean that the prescription chart does not leave the ward and remains with the medical record.

Ninety per cent of patients have no change in their medication during the latter stage of their inpatient stay and the initial supply for their discharge is thus ready on the ward for the patient to take home.

The use of lockers has:

- removed the need to re-supply medicines when a patient moves to another ward;

- speeded up medicines administration rounds;

- almost eliminated medicine and patient selection errors (only one reported instance on 10 wards in the first 12 months of the initiative); and

- reduced the amount of medicines stored on wards and in the dispensary.

The initiative also aimed to improve the quality of the information about a patient's therapy at admission, during the inpatient stay and upon discharge to GPs. The quality and accuracy of information at admission was improved by having patients' own medicines available for the admitting staff to see. The technicians' ward-prepared medicines sheet provided dispensary staff with a full record of current therapy to refer to when dealing with additional supply requests or other queries about a patient's therapy. Improving the quality of information to GPs on discharge has focused on those groups of patients that are most at risk if their treatment reverts to that in place before admission.

The next steps

The trust is in a good position to implement patient self-medication; patient lockers are in place and nursing staff have welcomed the fact that medicine administration rounds are now quicker. The more effective use of pharmacists' time also means more resources are available to train nurses in facilitating self-administration.

Lessons

- The need to shift resources from non-pay to pay budgets to fund innovation;

- The need to work across the whole health economy; and

- The need to adopt innovation that is tried and tested, and supported by research evidence.

Financial planning

92. The fourth strategic challenge for trust boards is to provide effective financial planning and control.

Current annual budgeting arrangements

93. In many hospitals, finance directors find it impossible to produce a balanced budget with the money available at the start of the year. Most hospitals therefore overspend their medicines budgets [EXHIBIT 14]. In many cases, finance directors have to rely on slippage from other budgets to offset the overspend on medicines.

94. When original budgets are constantly overspent in this way, it is a sure sign that the original budget was wrong. Medicines cost pressures are now being made more explicit through the work of NICE, and some trusts are working across the health economy to identify the full extent and necessary funding of future costs pressures [CASE STUDY 5, overleaf].

95. Many of the proposals contained in this report require an initial investment to improve the quality of medicines management and reduce the costs of medication errors. A characteristic of trusts that have achieved significant progress is the willingness of the trust to transfer money from non-pay to pay budgets. For example, investment in clinical pharmacy services needs initial funding, but a good clinical pharmacist will save his or her salary in the same financial year.

EXHIBIT 14

Comparison of trusts' outturn expenditure on medicines and original budgets

One in three trusts overspent their 2000/01 medicines budgets by more than 10 per cent.

N=157

Source: Audit Commission acute hospitals portfolio data

Number of trusts

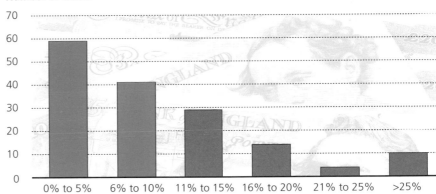

Percentage overspend 2000/01 (original budget vs. outturn)

Identifying future medicines cost pressures

To improve annual budget-setting at Salford Hospitals, directorate pharmacists and their clinical colleagues prepare an assessment of future medicines cost pressures and develop a planned approach to the introduction of new medicines in consultation with health authorities and local PCG/Ts.

The assessment identifies existing medicines that have an identified change in use or a change in clinical practice that will generate future cost pressures.

Arrangements for in-year cost pressures are agreed between commissioners and providers on the basis of 'shared-risk'.

Example of medicines cost pressures 2000/01 – Salford Hospitals NHS Trust

SPECIALTY	CLINICAL PROBLEM	MEDICINES REQUIRED	UNAVOIDABLE £	HARD TO AVOID £	DESIRABLE £
General	Microbial resistance	Synercid/Linezolid	60,000		
	IV Administration	Pre-made syringes/ minibags EL(97)52	50,000		
	DVT and PE Homecare	Low molecular weight heparins to reduce bed stay		20,000	
	Epilepsy	Oxcarbazepine		1,000	
	Trigeminal Neuralgia	Gabapentin		2,000	
	Anaemia in dialysis patients	Erythropoietin – virement to hospitals		80,000	
	Hepatitis C	Ribavirin and Interferon alpha	36,000		
Dermatology	Psoriasis	Infliximab	80,000		
Cardio/Pulmonary	PCTA/stent medicines	Clopidogrel – Cardiology	10,000		
	PCTA/stent medicines	Abciximab – Cardiology	100,000		
	Cardiopathies	Glycoprotein iib/iiia blockers – NICE guidance	250,000		
	Asthma	Chimeric monoclonal antibodies	450,000		
Anaesthesia	Muscle relaxation	Rapacuronium			Not known
	Total IV anaesthesia	Propofol			25,000
Palliative Care	Palliative Care	Specialist medicines		25,000	
Surgery	Endometriosis	Mirena – unlicensed use			4,080
	Premature infants	Palivizumab – prevention of RSV			20,000
	Urology – CA bladder	BCG for irrigation		10,000	
TOTALS			**586,000**	**588,000**	**50,080**

Source: Salford Hospitals NHS Trust

Pharmacists need to... work closely with PASA and the procurement professionals in their trusts to develop strategic partnerships with key suppliers.

Procurement

96. A number of regional contracts for medicines between the NHS Purchasing and Supply Agency (PASA) (and its predecessors) and suppliers has long been established. These cover about 60 per cent of product lines and seek to aggregate NHS purchasing power.

97. However, regional contracts have, to some extent, been weakened by hospitals renegotiating them in order to gain short-term price advantage. Suppliers have in all probability anticipated the likelihood of local re-negotiations when making tender offers to the NHS.

98. A Ministerial letter sent to trusts in January 2001 makes clear the Government's view about procurement in England. It wants:

- procurement and supplies issues are to be considered regularly by trust boards;
- more of trusts' non-pay expenditure, including medicines, are to be covered in a cohesive strategy; and
- a united NHS front presented to suppliers – contracts established by the PASA should be adhered to, not ignored or re-negotiated.

99. For medicines that are not covered by regional contracts, pharmacists in both English and Welsh trusts have a strong track-record of working in consortia, using their purchasing power and commitment to contract volume to reduce prices.

100. However, while prices are strongly controlled, there is patchy performance in other aspects of supply: hospitals in London are currently experiencing particularly poor performance from wholesalers in terms of late deliveries and partially-filled orders, although in Wales wholesaler performance is much better. Across the country, there are also few examples of the use of consignment stocks or of using suppliers to help with management information on performance and use.

101. Pharmacists need to build on their procurement expertise and work closely with PASA and the procurement professionals in their trusts to develop strategic partnerships with key suppliers. These arrangements should seek to ensure that both buyers and sellers work together to take advantage of the significant opportunities that exist to reduce process and transaction costs in the whole medicines supply chain.

102. Greater use of technology would also reduce process costs. Work by PASA has found that moving from manual to electronic updating of contract details in hospitals reduces the time taken for this task from 20 staff days a year to two.

103. Both the Association of the British Pharmaceutical Industry and PASA are aware of the opportunities to improve service standards and reduce total supply chain costs, and should work with trusts to deliver them.

104. However, as previously noted, it is not known how much of the variation in prescribing activity between hospitals is explained by differences in the age and medical condition of the patients treated. The current absence of any arrangement to aggregate local data associated with prescribing, purchasing and supplying medicines to a national level will limit the effectiveness of NHS procurement in general and the potential benefits offered by e-commerce in particular.

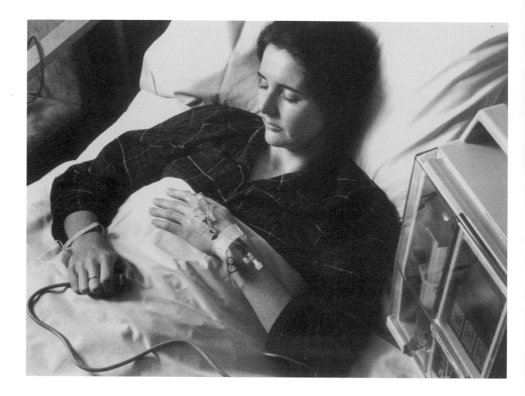

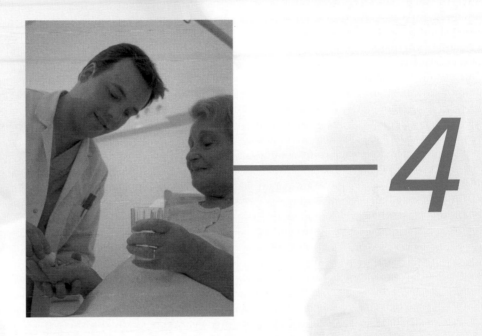

4

Obstacles to Progress and How to Overcome Them

In order to meet the strategic challenges presented by the
medicines management agenda, hospitals need to elevate
the status of some pharmacy services to focus their attention
on patient care, address staff recruitment and retention
problems, and invest in computer technology to reduce
risk to patients.

105. Three main obstacles need to be overcome in order to meet the strategic challenges that are described in the previous chapter. They are:

• the current low status of some hospital pharmacy services;

• staff recruitment and retention problems; and

• the need to introduce computer technology.

The status of pharmacy services

106. The importance of the pharmacist's role needs greater recognition outside the profession, especially at board level; and sometimes within the profession.

Attitudes outside the profession

107. Research evidence that supports innovation is overwhelming in areas such as:

• pro-active care on admission;

• re-engineering supply through the use of original pack dispensing;

• medication review clinics;

• better use of pharmacy technicians;

• development of pro-active clinical pharmacy services;

• self-administration of medicines by patients;

• pharmacist prescribing; and

• the use of IT and automation.

108. But not enough trust boards have acted on this evidence and considered sufficiently the link between medicines management and effective clinical governance.

...trust boards often appoint new consultants without reference to the effect that their additional workload will have on pharmacy services.

109. There is also a tendency to regard pharmacy merely as another support service, rather than one that is absolutely vital to the quality of patient care. For example, trust boards often appoint new consultants without reference to the effect that their additional workload will have on pharmacy services.

110. At the hospitals visited, auditors reviewed the background papers making the case to trust boards for the appointment of consultants, but in only one case out of twenty was there explicit reference to the impact that the new consultant would have on the demand for pharmacy services.

111. The NHS is seeking to recruit 7,500 new consultants and 20,000 nurses as part of the NHS Plan (Ref. 3). It is important that boards make provision for the impact that they will have on pharmacy services.

112. Medicines management is so vital to the quality of patient care that its status, and the status of hospital chief pharmacists, need to be reviewed in many hospitals. At the hospitals visited, greatest progress in delivering the strategic challenges outlined in this report had been achieved where the head of the pharmacy service held a position equivalent to that of a clinical director.

113. The introduction of directors of pharmacy would also open up greater career opportunities further down the organisational hierarchy and would help to reverse the exodus of pharmacists from the hospital service.

Attitudes within the profession

114. Attitudes also need to change within the profession. In some pharmacy services, there is an inherent conservatism and a need to 'market' pharmacy positively to senior management. If trusts are to optimise the use of medicines, pharmacy needs to be a core clinical function.

115. Excellent pharmacy services are characterised by:

- a chief pharmacist with the necessary strategic vision and political skills to ensure that pharmacy services are given due prominence with its key 'customers';

- pharmacists with the necessary skills of persuasion and negotiation, to manage working relationships with their clinical colleagues; and

- recognition by the trust board that pharmacy is first and foremost a clinical service.

116. The introduction of the four-year master's degree for pharmacists will improve the quality of clinical education, but developing management and influencing skills also needs attention, both at a professional level and through on-the-job training and coaching.

117. The Royal Pharmaceutical Society of Great Britain (RPSGB) also has a major role to play in equipping a new generation of pharmacists for enhanced clinical and managerial roles. The Society therefore should review the adequacy of its current support for hospital pharmacists' education and training; continuing professional development; professional competence and performance; and its workforce planning arrangements.

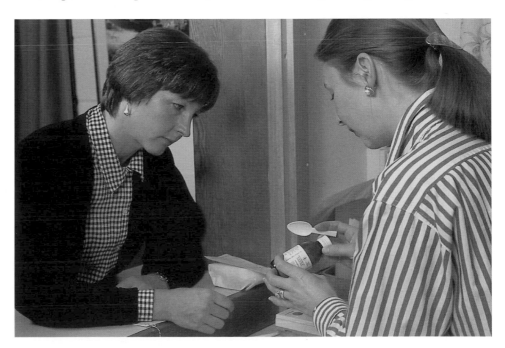

Staffing

Staff shortages

118. The number of hospital pharmacy staff has increased by 25 per cent in the last five years. Most of the increase is due to a growth in pharmacy technicians [**EXHIBIT 15**].

119. Despite these increases, 15 per cent of pharmacy posts are still vacant.[1] One-half of the hospitals in the UK are unable to provide all their intended pharmacy services because of staff shortages (Ref. 74). Overcoming these shortages in the short-term is unlikely – supply has been curtailed by increasing the length of pharmacy undergraduate courses to four years. In 2000/01, there were very few new pharmacy graduates going on to take their pre-registration training year, so in 2001/02 there will be very few newly qualified pharmacists.

120. The effect of these continued shortages is exacerbated by growing demand for pharmacy staff:

- demand for pharmacists from outside the hospital sector;
- increases in demand from traditional workload areas;
- increases in demand from new services; and
- the need to increase pharmacy operating hours.

Demand for pharmacists from outside the hospital sector

121. Demand for pharmacists has been increased by the requirement that all PCG/Ts or LHGs have a pharmaceutical adviser. There is also demand from private sector pharmacies, particularly the supermarket chains, some of whom are able to attract pharmacists because of better pay and conditions.

---

1   National hospital pharmacy vacancy survey 1999, conducted by the NHS Pharmacy Education and Development Committee.

EXHIBIT 15

Whole time equivalent staff employed in hospital pharmacies

The number of hospital pharmacy staff has increased by about 25 per cent in the last five years.

Source: Audit Commission analysis of data supplied by the DoH

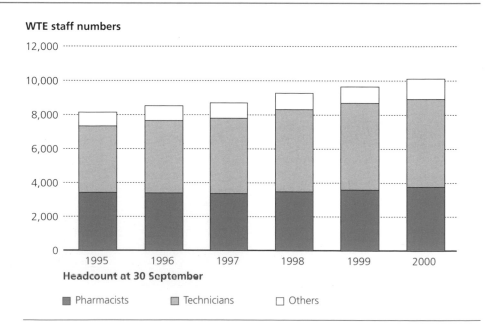

WTE staff numbers

Headcount at 30 September

■ Pharmacists   ■ Technicians   □ Others

Increases in demand from traditional service areas

122. The number of inpatient episodes has increased by about 10 per cent in the last five years, and the number of prescriptions written per patient has also increased. This has had an effect on traditional pharmacy services, such as dispensing.

Demand from new services

123. Workload pressures also stem from the demand to extend pharmacists' clinical roles (Ref. 75). For example, in outpatient services, there are demands for pharmacists to run anticoagulant clinics and therapeutic drug monitoring clinics. Pharmacists are also assuming responsibility for managing inpatient anticoagulation and aspects of dose adjustment for some shared care medicines.

124. Supplying medicines under patient group directions, as set out in the NHS Plan, will enhance the role of pharmacists in the multi-disciplinary clinical team, both as trainers and as clinicians (Ref. 3). Studies have shown that pharmacist involvement produces benefits in patient outcomes, improves the quality of doctors' prescribing and saves money (Ref. 76). As well as taking these steps, trusts should anticipate possible changes to the Medicines Act that will allow pharmacists to act as full independent prescribers.

125. Schemes such as pharmacist prescribing will force pharmacists away from their traditional, re-active model of prescription review to adopting a more pro-active role. Currently, pharmacists spend a significant amount of time annotating patients' prescription charts. However, these interventions take place, on average, 48 hours after the patient has been given their medication **[EXHIBIT 16]** (Ref. 77). Since some errors are potentially life-threatening, it is clear that a pro-active approach would be safer for patients. However, introducing pro-active rather than re-active pharmacy services will place further demands on pharmacists' time.

EXHIBIT 16

Average time between prescription and identification/correction of a problem

There are significant delays between prescription errors and intervention.

Category of error

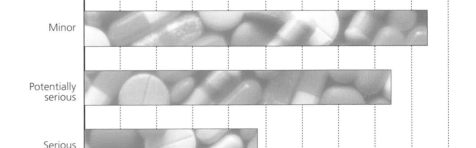

Average hours between prescription and intervention

Source: Ref. 77

...an extension of service hours is unavoidable if hospitals are to deliver all aspects of pharmaceutical care uniformly...

126. On all fronts, pharmacy services should be asked to provide a more pro-active approach. Prescriptions should be reviewed on or as soon after admission as possible; reviews of patients' own medicines are needed; and there is a growing demand for pharmacy involvement in discharge planning (Ref. 78).

127. The clinical role of pharmacists will further increase with the likely growth of pharmacist prescribing (expected following the provisions of the 2001 *Health and Social Care Act*) (Ref. 79).

128. The quality of patient care and cost-effectiveness of medicines use can be achieved by enhancing the role of the clinical pharmacist in the multi-disciplinary team. Enhancing their role would also reduce the workload of doctors in training. Such schemes have been found to improve the quality of doctors' prescribing, as well as saving money (Ref. 80).

The need to extend pharmacy operating hours

129. Finally, workload demands are placed on pharmacy services by the need to move away from the traditional model of a 9 to 5, Monday to Friday service.

130. Extending the pharmacy service's operating hours makes sense given the time of day when prescriptions are written. Up to one-half of inpatient prescriptions are written outside the traditional 9 to 5 weekday working hours [EXHIBIT 17]; over the weekend, 77 per cent of prescriptions are written outside the traditional three-hour Saturday service (9am–12 noon) (Ref. 81). Thus, an extension of service hours is unavoidable if hospitals are to deliver all aspects of pharmaceutical care uniformly to all patients.

131. Moving to a 24-hour, seven days a week service would be impractical in most hospitals on cost grounds. However, extending ward-based services into the early evening and at weekends appears logical.

132. The pattern of hospital work also means that adequate arrangements must be in place for on-call medicines information services. The opportunities afforded by computer technology should enable more of these services to be provided off-site and out of hours in order to minimise cost.

EXHIBIT 17

The time of day that prescriptions are written

Prescriptions are written around the clock.

Number of items dispensed

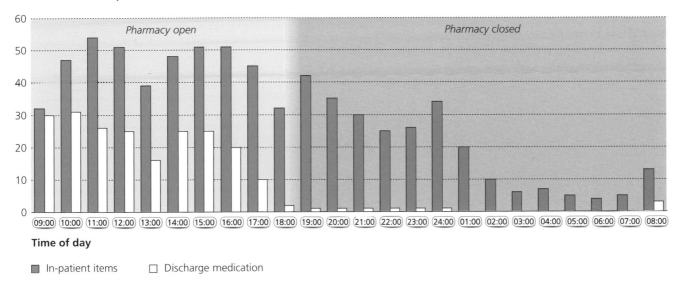

Source: Audit Commission (surveys from four study sites, based on the research model in ref. 81)

Tackling staff shortages

133. Trusts can tackle staff shortages by investing a sustained effort in the following areas:

- introducing more flexible working patterns;
- re-engineering pharmacy services;
- redesigning and enriching jobs;
- introducing automation;
- providing administrative support; and
- reviewing make or buy decisions.

Introducing more flexible working patterns

134. Some trusts need to offer more attractive remuneration packages and flexible working conditions to attract and retain pharmacists. Women make up 68 per cent of the pharmacy workforce and 70 per cent of them are under 40 years old (Ref. 82). Delivering the NHS's *Improved Working Lives Directive* is highly important to meet their needs (Ref. 83).

Re-engineering pharmacy services

135. The principal objective of a re-engineered service is to put pharmacists closer to patients as this is where they add the greatest value. Trusts should review the tasks that are being undertaken by pharmacists with a view to ensuring that this objective is met, while activities like dispensing are automated. Revision and expansion of the pharmacy technician and pharmacy assistant roles need to play a major part in this strategy, provided that proper competency assessments are established and adhered to [BOX I].

136. The role of the pharmacy technician is now so pivotal to hospital pharmacy services that the RPSGB should consider the formal registration of pharmacy technicians.

Job design and enrichment

137. Studies of staff turnover have found that there is wide and unexplained variation in turnover between trusts in similar geographic locations (Ref. 84). Although local and national economic factors play their part, more than one-half of the variation is explained by differences in the way that trusts manage their staff. At the trusts visited, it was notable that while most reported recruitment and retention problems, those at the leading edge of medicines management practice reported that their services were not adversely affected by recruitment and retention problems.

BOX I

Main roles in pharmacy services

Pharmacists' key roles

- Prescribing (once the provisions of the Health & Social Care Act are implemented)
- Clinical governance
- Preparing guidelines of clinical care
- Ward rounds
- Teaching
- Reviewing whole health economy prescribing
- Running certain clinics
- Medicines information services

Pharmacy technicians' key roles

- Clinical pharmacy services within agreed guidelines
- Procurement of medicines
- All aspects of supply and dispensing of medicines
- Educating for concordance
- Checking patients' own medication

Pharmacy assistant key roles

- Supply of medicines – inpatient and stock dispensing (with checking by a pharmacy technician)

- Regular top-up service to wards and theatres
- Dispensary and aseptic support

Services that could be supported by non-pharmacy staff

- Business planning
- Performance management
- Data management
- Some aspects of procurement

Services that could be supported by automation

- Dispensing

138. Enriching the work of technicians is particularly important if staff are to be retained. Some pharmacy services make extensive use of pharmacy technicians to undertake work that was hitherto the preserve of registered staff, such as procurement, supply and dispensing functions. University courses are also now available to train technicians in clinical pharmacy roles.

Automation

139. Staff can also be released through automated dispensing. Robotic systems release staff for patient-centred services, and reduce dispensing errors [CASE STUDY 6] (Ref. 85).

140. Few trusts are likely to have the capital or the expertise to invest in these systems, and there seems little sense in trusts individually specifying different systems. Economy of scale, and standardisation of systems and barcodes, could be achieved if the DoH and the National Assembly jointly commissioned a national specification for automated dispensing. The provision of earmarked funds to roll-out the introduction of these systems to all large acute hospitals might also be considered in light of the improvements they offer.

Robotic systems release staff for patient-centred services, and reduce dispensing errors.

CASE STUDY 6

Wirral Hospitals NHS Trust's robotic dispensing system

Wirral Hospital installed a robotic dispensing system in January 2001, at a cost of £300,000. The business case was approved by the board on the grounds that the system would reduce dispensing error rates and release staff to manage medicines at ward level.

Items are bar-coded and selected for dispensing via remote terminals. The systems covers 77 per cent of medicines items, handling mainly items in whole containers.

The system dispenses between 900 and 1,200 items each day.

The benefits of the system include:

- dispensary turnaround times have been reduced;
- reported dispensing errors reduced from 19 per 100,000 to 7 per 100,000;
- ordering processes are simplified;
- improved reliability of service;
- more efficient use of staff – three whole time equivalent pharmacy technicians have been released to support direct patient care;
- reduced staff down time;
- potential use of consignment stocking;
- 70 per cent less shelving needed; and
- floor space required has been reduced by one-half.

Managerial support

141. Some managerial and administrative tasks that are undertaken by qualified pharmacists could be undertaken equally well by non-clinical staff. General managers and administrative staff should be used for tasks that they can perform, such as business planning, performance review and data management.

Make or buy decisions

142. The DoH's Controls Assurance Standards for Medicines Management acknowledges that aseptic dispensing is an increasing and demanding activity for pharmacy services (Ref. 1). Some NHS manufacturing capacity is also needed to provide medicines that are not commercially available. However, boards should always consider whether collaboration with other trusts for the provision of common aseptically prepared items and manufacturing is a viable alternative to individual trusts investing in these services. Such collaboration may be a way to release pharmacy staff and capital for investment in other activities.

Computer technology

143. Computerised prescribing linked with electronic health records will radically alter the way in which care is provided and will deliver significant improvements in the quality of patient care (Ref. 86). The introduction of these systems, which ultimately need to be accessible by primary care and other hospitals, is vital to provide access to common clinical data. It is one of the biggest challenges currently facing the NHS.

144. The Information for Health strategy expects 35 per cent of trusts to have installed electronic patient record systems (including the reporting of results and prescribing) by 2002, and all trusts by 2005 (Ref. 87). The strategy provided £60 million (about £600,000 for an average health authority) to which a further £250 million is provided in the NHS Plan. However, the funds are not ringfenced, so some trusts have spent less because of competing priorities and deficits, and generally progress is extremely slow.

145. These systems have been introduced in only a few hospitals. Two trusts that have introduced them successfully share a number of common attributes [CASE STUDY 7].

Introducing electronic patient records – Burton on Trent Hospitals and Wirral Hospitals

Background

A major source of risk and avoidable costs in hospitals stems from inadequate patient records. Patient care is jeopardised by inaccurate, illegible or lost paper records; professionals' time is wasted and errors in diagnosis and treatment are made because accurate information is not available at the time decisions are made.

The technology to deliver electronic patient records (EPR) in hospitals has been around for more than 10 years but few hospitals have been successful in managing the changes that are necessary to implement these systems.

Organisational context

Stability

Unlike most NHS trusts, Burton and Wirral have avoided significant organisational change over the last 10 years – there has been no significant merger activity.

Both trusts have a comparative organisational simplicity – both are geographically isolated with clear catchment populations, referral lines into primary care and links with their health authorities. This has created an environment that to some extent insulates both trusts from 'politicisation', competition and some would say outside interference.

Both trusts are of a manageable size. Some hold the view that change is easier in organisations of this scale, because senior people can 'see across the organisation'

and are therefore more prepared to take managerial risk. The sheer size and organisational complexity of the larger teaching trusts may make informal networking and commitment building difficult.

There was extraordinary stability in key personnel at both trusts. Wirral kept the same chief executive and chief pharmacist throughout the 1990s; Burton also had the same chief pharmacist, and promoted their medical director into the chief executive's post when it became vacant. Both retained the same core of lead consultants. This consistency is regarded as vital in maintaining direction and ensuring high priority for EPR implementation.

Funding

Both EPR projects were pump-primed with additional ear-marked funds – Wirral was a first wave, and Burton a second wave Resource Management Initiative site.

'Marketing' the system objectives

In both trusts, the systems were designed and 'marketed' to improve the process of patient care, not to save money. The benefits were described in terms of reduced patient risk and improved clinical audit. Although there are secondary financial benefits, through reduced process costs and better use of medicines, these benefits were never seen as central to either project. This approach helped to ensure professional support.

Providing the capacity to deliver change

Both organisations created managerial slack to invest in the change process. Both projects were led by small, multidisciplinary project boards of 5 or 6 individuals. Large, representative working parties were avoided. The project boards were professionally-led, not dominated by finance or technical staff.

Change takes time

There was an acceptance in both organisations that change would take a significant amount of time because the work involved re-engineering the way that doctors, nurses and other clinicians work. The procurement processes alone took two years. This commitment at board level helped to insulate the change processes from competing priorities.

Clear milestones

Both projects had clear milestones, breaking the project down into manageable pieces. Both trusts rolled their projects out on to wards where they expected the most support from the staff involved, and both were willing to retreat and retrench in the face of opposition.

Measuring change

Both trusts (perhaps by virtue of the 'scientific' management style of doctors and pharmacists) collected baseline data on key indicators to demonstrate benefits and calibrate the success of the new systems. Data included measuring (reduced)

cont./

CASE STUDY 7 (cont.)

medication errors, speed of test results, discharge delays, and additional time spent with patients. Collecting the baseline data helped to maintain commitment to the projects at board level, and to demonstrate their value in the face of competing priorities.

Making change stick

Introducing EPR and electronic prescribing (EP) radically changes the way that patient care is delivered – once paper systems are abandoned there is no 'going back.' This places a premium (and cost) on training new staff. Temporary staff – particularly locum doctors – are unable to work without full training in the systems. Potential new consultants are asked to confirm at interview that they would work with EPRs and EP, and are not appointed if they are unwilling.

Wider lessons

On the evidence of this case study, the key ingredients that lead to success in implementing EPR are:

- staff and organisational stability;

- insulating the change process;

- accepting that change takes time; and

- collecting data to calibrate progress.

146. Computer technology is not an optional extra but a fundamental part of the modernisation agenda on which to build other changes required by the *NHS Plan* and *Improving Health in Wales*, including the implementation of effective clinical governance (Refs. 3 and 4). Technology is also the way to release scarce pharmacy resources into direct patient care [EXHIBIT 18].

EXHIBIT 18

How pharmacists' time is spent

Pharmacists in trusts with automated dispensing and electronic prescribing systems are able to devote more time to direct patient care.

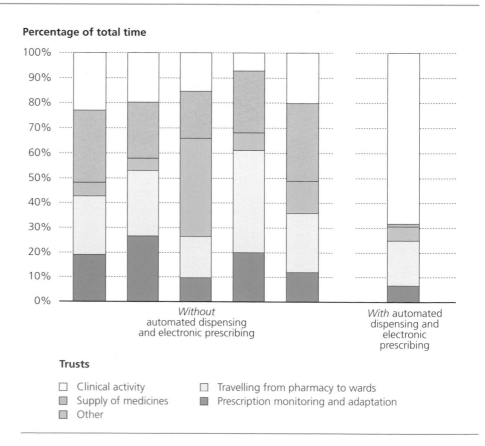

Percentage of total time

Without automated dispensing and electronic prescribing

With automated dispensing and electronic prescribing

Trusts

- ☐ Clinical activity
- ☐ Travelling from pharmacy to wards
- ◼ Supply of medicines
- ◼ Prescription monitoring and adaptation
- ◼ Other

Source: Ref 92

147. Achieving the targets that are set out in the Information Management and Technology (IM and T) strategy in respect of electronic health records and electronic prescribing systems is a tall order given the current state of development in most trusts (Ref. 88). Only one in three executive directors surveyed said that their trusts had clear plans to introduce these systems. On current progress it is likely that less than 10 per cent of trusts will meet the 2005 deadline.

148. Urgent action is needed to put the IM and T strategy back on course. A standard national system for coding medicines across the NHS is required to support the introduction of electronic prescribing and electronic health records. Earmarked funds and expertise should be considered, as well as central guidance on systems specifications, screen layouts and coding structures. Such a centralised approach would prevent unnecessary duplication of effort, provide economy of scale in procurement and would make working with the NHS in this area a more attractive proposition to suppliers of IT and software systems.

Urgent action is needed to put the IM and T strategy back on course.

149. As well as the significant cost of the computers and software, the introduction of new systems will fundamentally alter the way that doctors, nurses and pharmacists work together to deliver patient care. Many trusts will need support and guidance in the organisational development aspects of introducing these new technologies.

150. The cost of introducing IT and software to deliver electronic health records and electronic prescribing systems to a typical hospital is in the region of £2 million, with £500,000 annual running costs. Much of the money needed is already available in the provisions of the IM and T strategy, and its investment would be recouped quickly by eliminating a large proportion of the £500 million spent each year on treating patients who are harmed by medication errors and adverse reactions.

151. A strongly centralised strategy runs directly counter to the government's philosophy of decentralisation, expressed in *Shifting the Balance of Power within the NHS* (Ref. 89). Nevertheless, it is an option that merits urgent and serious consideration.

5

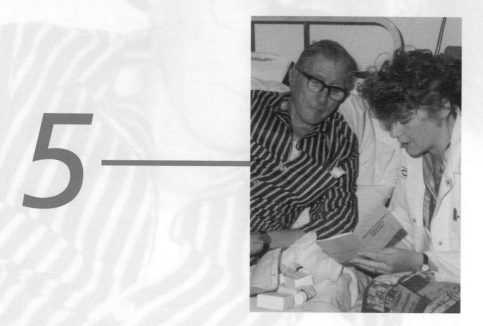

The Way Forward

Urgent action and investment are needed in many hospitals
to bring medicines management arrangements up to the
level of the best. The risks of not acting are substantial, both
in terms of the quality of patient care and the costs to the
NHS. Maintaining the status quo is not a viable option.

The NHS Plan

152. The main principles that underpin the NHS Plan are to:

- re-shape care around the patient;
- improve quality; and
- make better use of NHS staff.

153. *Pharmacy in the Future – Implementing the NHS Plan* covers issues that are relevant to medicines management (Ref. 9). It envisages some radical shifts in job design [BOX J] and support for medicines management [BOX K].

BOX J

Principal responsibilities in medicines management implied by the NHS Plan

JOB	TRADITIONAL MODEL	NEW MODEL (?)
Diagnose disease state	Doctor	Doctor/pharmacist/nurse
Decide therapy	Doctor/pharmacist	Doctor/pharmacist/nurse/patient
Supply the therapy	Pharmacist	Nurses (under guidelines)
Administer the therapy	Nurses	Patients

BOX K

The relevance of the NHS Plan to medicines management

NHS PLAN COMMITMENT	RELEVANCE TO MEDICINES MANAGEMENT
The 'expert patient' programme will be extended – NICE will publish patient-friendly versions of clinical guidelines	Argues for greater use of patients' own medicines; and self-medication
Breaking down the barriers between staff (£10m for increased nurse prescribing)	Qualified nurses, midwives, therapists and pharmacists will be empowered to undertake a broader range of clinical tasks, including for some prescribing medicines and for the majority supplying medicines under Patient Group Directions
£250m for IT	Integrated electronic patient records are very important to improving the quality of medicines management services – for example, improving links across healthcare organisations
£140m to ensure that all professional staff are supported in keeping their skills up-to-date and to provide access to learning for all NHS staff without a professional qualification	Presents an opportunity to increase the skills of administrative staff and technicians and so release pharmacists for professional work
£30m to boost childcare	One-half of all hospital pharmacists are women. Family-friendly policies would ease recruitment and retention problems

What should trust boards do?

...trust boards will need to invest in computer systems and automation in order to release pharmacy staff resources into direct patient services.

154. Action is required on several fronts to deliver better medicines management. The DoH has much to do in delivering the agenda set out in *Building a Safer NHS for Patients*, and the IM and T strategy (Refs. 6 and 88). The pharmaceutical supply industry, too, should also be taking a more pro-active role: it shares the same interests as the NHS in ensuring the efficacy of medicines; in eliminating unnecessary supply-chain costs; and in improving patients' compliance with medication.

155. But this report has been mainly about what trust boards must do. It is important not to underestimate the scale of the task that they face in delivering the agenda that is described in this report. This is not through a lack of desire or interest but due to the time and staff required to lead and implement the changes.

156. The list of recommendations provides a challenging agenda for change. A systematic approach needs to be taken by each trust. They need to compare their current position against the recommendations of this report, then prioritise actions, plan, and monitor the outcomes. It is a daunting agenda, where a significant investment of money and effort is needed to secure progress. But the risks of not acting are substantial, both in terms of the quality of patient care and the costs to the NHS.

157. In particular, trust boards will need to invest in computer systems and automation in order to release pharmacy staff resources into direct patient services. Investment in training and development will also be needed to increase the knowledge base in order to provide comprehensive clinical pharmacy services.

The DoH medicines management framework

158. The DoH has emphasised its commitment to the importance of medicines management through the dissemination of its framework. The framework will indicate to trust boards where progress is needed locally in the following areas:

- senior management commitment;
- financial control;
- policy on the use of medicines;
- procurement;
- primary care interface;
- prescribing influence; and
- risk management.

159. A preliminary review of the framework returns suggests that, of the seven areas, senior management commitment is the one where significant improvement is needed.

160. Over the coming months, returns from the medicines management framework will be analysed in conjunction with returns to the Audit Commission's acute hospitals portfolio. The DoH should consider using this exercise to enable identification of Beacon Sites for medicines management. These trusts should then be funded to run open days that are aimed at board members. Dissemination of good practice in this way needs to be encouraged. A mechanism to make readily available advice, guidance and the experience of achieving the goals stated in this report would be beneficial to trusts.

Local audits

161. The Commission has collected quantitative data about acute hospitals' medicines management arrangements. Where analysis highlights shortcomings, the Commission's auditors will recommend in-depth reviews as part of their performance management audit. Auditors will then tailor the findings and recommendations of this report to local circumstances.

162. Local audits will supplement the DoH initiative and generate much-needed attention to raising the profile of medicines management. All trusts and health authorities should consider auditors' recommendations in the context of their overall responsibilities for clinical governance.

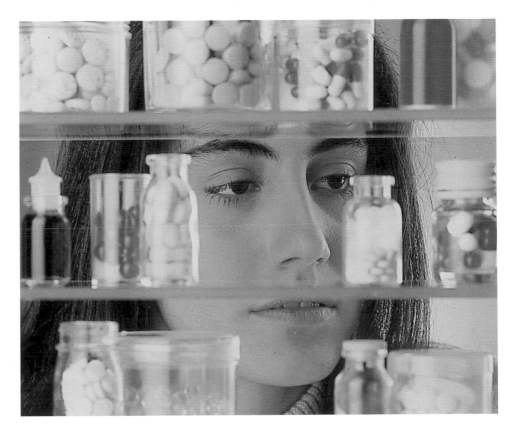

RECOMMENDATIONS

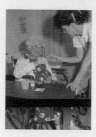

The terminology used in these recommendations is aimed at England; however, they are broadly consistent with the recommendations that are made in the the National Assembly's *Report of the Task and Finish Group on Prescribing* (Ref. 7).

For the Department of Health and the National Assembly for Wales

1 The establishment of standard nation-wide definitions and categories of medication errors and 'near-misses' should be an early priority for the new National Patient Safety Agency. Trusts should be required to adopt such systems as part of their clinical governance arrangements and should report progress in their annual reports, as well as reporting along the lines proposed in *Building a Safer NHS* (Ref. 6).
(Paragraph 36)

2 Following agreement of standard definitions and categories of medication errors, base-line audits should be undertaken with central funding at a representative sample of hospitals to calibrate the current situation in order that improvement targets can be set and their achievement monitored. Work should prioritise specialties with the highest likely risk.
(Paragraph 37)

3 National co-ordination of publicity posters should be considered to encourage patients to take their medicines into hospital with them.
(Paragraph 72)

4 The DoH and the National Assembly need to work with HM Customs and Excise to equalise tax treatments between hospital and community sectors and thus remove what is becoming an obstacle to best prescribing practice.
(Paragraph 90)

5 The DoH and the National Assembly should commission a specification for automated dispensary systems and consider the provision of earmarked funds to roll-out the introduction of these systems to all trusts.
(Paragraph 140)

6 A standard national system for the coding of medicines and barcodes should be introduced across the whole of the NHS to support the development of electronic prescribing systems and automated dispensing systems.
(Paragraphs 140 and 148)

7 Earmarked funds should be made available to enable trusts to comply with the targets that are set in the NHS IM and T strategy (Ref. 88). Central guidance on systems specification and screen layouts should be considered.
(Paragraph 148)

RECOMMENDATIONS

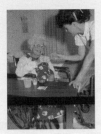

8 Trusts' medicines management framework returns should be analysed in conjunction with returns to the Audit Commission's acute hospitals portfolio. The DoH and the National Assembly should consider using this exercise to enable the identification of Beacon Sites for medicines management. These trusts should then be funded to run open days aimed at board members.
(Paragraph 160)

For the Royal Pharmaceutical Society of Great Britain

9 The RPSGB should review the adequacy of its current support for hospital pharmacists' education and training; continuing professional development; professional competence and performance; and its workforce planning arrangements.
(Paragraph 117)

10 The RPSGB should consider introducing the formal registration of pharmacy technicians.
(Paragraph 136)

For the NHS Purchasing and Supply Agency

11 PASA should consider establishing a national contract for the supply of patients' medicines lockers.
(Paragraph 80).

12 PASA should work with trusts and with the Association of the British Pharmaceutical Industry to examine and eliminate supply chain costs and improve wholesaler and supplier performance where necessary.
(Paragraphs 101 to 103)

For NHS trust boards

13 Trust boards should use the DoH's Medicines Management Framework in conjunction with the Audit Commission's diagnostic to review medicines management arrangements and develop local action plans (Ref. 2).
(Paragraph 23)

14 Medicines formularies should be agreed that are linked to joint care arrangements, clinical guidelines and NICE guidance.
(Paragraph 28)

15 Medicines management groups and DTCs should be made formally accountable to the trust board or to the clinical governance committee.
(Paragraph 28)

RECOMMENDATIONS

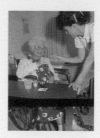

16 Risk management arrangements should be reviewed and 'fair blame' and 'near miss' reporting systems introduced.
(Paragraphs 44 to 45)

17 Trust boards and senior managers should seek regular assurance that actual clinical practice reflects agreed protocols – in particular, the practice of making-up aseptic preparations on hospital wards should be stopped.
(Paragraph 46)

18 Lead clinicians should ensure that the induction programme of all clinical staff provides adequate coverage of policies on prescribing practice, medicines administration and incident reporting. Monitoring of competencies in prescription and administration of medicines should be given high priority.
(Paragraphs 47 and 48)

19 Trusts should undertake reviews of pharmacy staffing levels and consider whether there are adequate resources to:

(i) provide for all aspects of clinical pharmacy services;

(ii) meet the demands of the NHS Plan in respect of new consultants and nurse prescribers;

(iii) take patients' medication histories; and

(iv) support dispensing for discharge schemes.

(Paragraphs 56 and 132)

20 Arrangements should be introduced for the use of patients' own medicines in hospital.
(Paragraphs 68 to 69)

21 Trust boards should call for a position statement on progress towards introducing self-administration of medicines and providing the necessary staff resource to maximise implementation.
(Paragraphs 72 to 82)

22 Original pack dispensing should be introduced in all appropriate areas immediately, using Department of Health guidance. Re-packaging of medicines from bulk should be stopped, wherever possible.
(Paragraphs 85 to 88)

23 The annual Service and Financial Framework round should include an assessment of future cost pressures from medicines, and a risk-sharing approach agreed between commissioners and providers.
(Paragraph 94 and Case study 5)

RECOMMENDATIONS

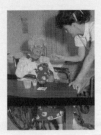

24 Transfer of money from non-pay to pay budgets should be considered in order to fund investment in pharmacy services.
(Paragraph 95)

25 Wherever possible, trusts should use PASA contracts for medicines.
(Paragraphs 96 to 98)

26 Pharmacists should work with procurement professionals in the development of strategic partnerships with the main suppliers.
(Paragraph 101)

27 Trusts should introduce electronic updating of supplier contract details.
(Paragraph 102)

28 Trust boards should always consider the impact on pharmacy services when appointing new consultants.
(Paragraph 111).

29 The role of chief pharmacist should be elevated to the equivalent of a clinical director and should be a member of the trust's management executive.
(Paragraph 112)

30 A review of pharmacy operating hours should be undertaken.
(Paragraph 130)

31 Recruitment and retention policies and practice should be reviewed to provide competitive working flexibilities and remuneration packages for pharmacists.
(Paragraph 134)

For Commissioners

32 Primary and secondary care should work together to consider limiting the practice of outpatient dispensing.
(Paragraphs 64 and 65)

33 Original pack dispensing should be introduced immediately.
(Paragraphs 95 to 97)

Appendix 1

Organisations visited

NHS bodies

Addenbrooke's Hospital

Airedale Hospitals and Health Authority

Birmingham Children's Hospital

Blackpool Victoria Hospitals

Burton Hospitals

Cardiothoracic Centre, Liverpool

East Riding NHS Trust and Health Authority

George Eliot Hospital

Guy's and St Thomas's

John Radcliffe Hospital

Kettering Hospital

Manchester Children's Hospital

Mid-Sussex NHS Trust

Milton Keynes Hospitals

North Birmingham Mental Health Trust

North Cheshire Hospitals

North Staffordshire Hospitals

Northumbria Healthcare

Oldham Hospitals

Plymouth Hospitals

QMC Nottingham

Salford Hospitals

South Warwickshire General Hospitals

United Lincolnshire NHS Trust

University Hospital of Wales

Wirral Hospitals

Regional meetings of chief pharmacists in Wales, West Midlands, South-East and London regions

Other organisations

Association of the British Pharmaceutical Industry

Boots

Centre for Practice and Policy, School of Pharmacy, University of London

Department of Health

Glaxo, SmithKline

National Prescribing Centre

NHS Purchasing and Supply Agency

Royal College of Nursing

Royal Pharmaceutical Society of Great Britain

Appendix 2

External advisors

The following individuals have supported the study team with advice and guidance:

Sue Ashwell	Kettering Hospitals NHS Trust
David Cousins	Derbyshire Royal Infirmary NHS Trust
Keith Farrar	Wirral Hospitals NHS Trust
John Farrell	Department of Health
Ray Fitzpatrick	North Staffordshire NHS Trust
Steve Freeborn	Royal Salford Hospitals NHS Trust
Kevin Guinness	Department of Health
Jeannette Howe	Deputy Chief Pharmacist, Department of Health
Maureen Milligan	Queen's Medical Centre, Nottingham
Eileen Neilson	Royal Pharmaceutical Society of Great Britain
Mike Pollard	North East Wales NHS Trust
Keith Ridge	Department of Health
David Roberts	University Hospital of Wales
David Scott	John Radcliffe Hospital, Oxford
Peter Sharott	Chelsea and Westminster Hospital NHS Trust
Ann Slee	Wirral Hospitals NHS Trust
Mike Spencer	University Hospital of Wales
Vic Standing	North Western Regional Pharmaceutical Advisor
Howard Stokoe	NHS Purchasing and Supply Agency
Debra Walker	National Prescribing Centre
Carwen Wynn-Howells	Chief Pharmacist, National Assembly for Wales

Study methodology

The work was undertaken principally by conducting observational reviews and audits at the organisations visited, by seeking expert opinion, and by analysing data and literature from secondary sources.

In addition, the Commission has collected data from all acute hospital trusts on aspects of their performance in delivering effective medicines management.

References

1. NHS Executive, *Controls Assurance Standards for Medicines Management*, Department of Health, 1999
2. Department of Health, *Medicines Management Framework*, 2001
3. Department of Health, *NHS Plan*, The Stationery Office, 2000
4. NHS Wales, *Improving Health in Wales*, The Stationery Office, 2001
5. Department of Health, *An Organisation with a Memory*, The Stationery Office, 2000
6. Department of Health, *Building a Safer NHS for Patients*, The Stationery Office, 2001
7. National Assembly for Wales, *Report of the Task and Finish Group on Prescribing*, 2000
8. Department of Health, HSC(99)/143, Review of NHS Procurement
9. Department of Health, *Pharmacy in the Future*, The Stationery Office, 2001
10. Department of Health, *National Service Framework for Older People*, The Stationery Office, 2001
11. Health Survey for England 1998, Vol 1: Findings
12. Cunningham G et al, Drug-related problems in elderly patients admitted to Tayside hospitals, methods for prevention and subsequent reassessment. *Age and Ageing*, 1997; 26:375–382
13. Mannesse CK et al, Adverse drug reactions in elderly patients as a contributing factor for hospital admission: cross-sectional study. *British Medical Journal* 1997; 315:1057–1058
14. Mannesse CK et al, Contribution of adverse drug reactions to hospital admission of older patients. *Age and Ageing*, 2000; 29:35–39
15. Royal Pharmaceutical Society of Great Britain, *National Sentinel Clinical Audit of Evidence-Based Prescribing for Older People*, Royal College of Physicians, 2000
16. Duggan C et al, Reducing adverse prescribing discrepancies following hospital discharge. *International Journal of Pharmacy Practice* 1998; 6:77–82
17. Duffin et al, An investigation into medication changes initiated in general practice after patients are discharged from hospital. *Pharmaceutical Journal*, 1998; 261(Suppl.):R32
18. Miller EFR et al, The development and validation of a hospital readmissions predictive model. *Pharmaceutical Journal*, 2000; 265:R55
19. Chu LW and Pei CK, Risk factors for early hospital re-admission in elderly patients, *Gerontology*, 1999; 45:220–226
20. Health Act 1999, The Stationery Office

21. Lesar TS, Briceland LL, Delcoure K, Parmalee JC, Masta-Gornic V, Pohl H, Medication prescribing errors in a teaching hospital. *Journal of the American Medical Association,* 1990; 263:2329–34.

22. Koren G, Barzilay Z, Greenwald M, Tenfold errors in administration of drug doses: a neglected iatrogenic disease in pediatrics. *Pediatrics,* 1986; 77:848–9

23. Allan EL, Barker KN, Fundamentals of medication error research. *American Journal of Hospital Pharmacy,* 1990; 47:555–71

24. Phillips DP et al, Increase in US medication error deaths between 1983 and 1993, *Lancet,* 1998; 351:643–44

25. Ferner RE, Whittington RM, Coroner's cases of death due to errors in prescribing or giving medicines or to adverse drug reactions: Birmingham 1986-1991. *Journal of the Royal Society of Medicine* 1994; 87:145–8

26. Bates DW, Cullen DJ, Laird N, Petersen LA, Small SD, Servi D et al, Incidence of adverse drug events and potential adverse drug events. Implications for prevention. *Journal of the American Medical Association,* 1995; 274:29–34

27. Vincent C et al, Adverse events in British hospitals: preliminary retrospective record review. *British Medical Journal,* 2001; 322:517–519

28. Department of Health, *The Prevention of Intrathecal Medication Errors,* 2001

29. Toft B, *External Inquiry into the adverse incident that occurred at Queen's Medical Centre, Nottingham,* 4th January 2001, Department of Health, 2001

30. Alberti KGMM, Medical errors: a common problem, *British Medical Journal;* 322:501–502

31. Woods K, *The Prevention of Intrathecal Medication Errors – A report to the Chief Medical Officer,* Department of Health, April 2001

32. Orton DI and Cruzelier JH, Adverse changes in mood and cognitive performance in house officers after night duty, *British Medical Journal,* 1989; 281:21–23

33. Firth-Cozens J, Stress, psychological problems and clinical performance. In Vincent, C et al, (ed.) *Medical Accidents.* Oxford: OUP, 1993:131–149

34. Johnson D, How the Atlantic Barons Learnt Teamwork, *British Medical Journal,* 2001; 322:563

35. Toft B, *External Inquiry into the adverse incident that occurred at Queen's Medical Centre, Nottingham,* 4th January 2001, Department of Health, 2001

36. Cousins D, Presentation to the European Association of Hospital Pharmacy Congress, Amsterdam, March 2001

37. Leape LL, Brennan TA, Laird N, Lawthers AG, Localio AR, Barnes BA et al, The nature of adverse events in hospitalized patients: results of the Harvard medical practice study II. *New England Journal of Medicine*, 1991; 324:377–384

38. Bates DW, Cullen DJ, Laird N, Petersen LA, Small SD, Servi D et al, Incidence of adverse drug events and potential adverse drug events: implications for prevention. *Journal of the American Medical Association*, 1995; 274:29–34

39. Ferner RE, Errors in prescribing and giving drugs. *Journal of the Medical Defence Union*, 1992; 8:60–63

40. Leape LL, Bates DW, Cullen DJ, Cooper J, Demonaco HJ, Gallivan T et al, Systems analysis of adverse drug events. *Journal of the American Medical Association*, 1995; 274: 35–43

41. Lesar TS, Briceland L, Stein DS, Factors related to errors in medication prescribing. *Journal of the American Medical Association*, 1997; 277: 312–317

42. Bates DW, Boyle DL, Vander Vliet M, Schneider J, Leape L, Relationship between medication errors and adverse drug events. *Journal of General International Medicine*, 1995; 10:199–205

43. Wyatt J, Walton R, Computer based prescribing: improves decision making and reduces costs. *British Medical Journal*, 1995; 311:1181–1182

44. Schiff GD, Rucker TD, Computerized prescribing: building the electronic infrastructure for better medication usage. *Journal of the American Medical Association*, 1998; 279:1024–1029

45. Johnston ME, Langton KB, Haynes RB, Mathieu A, Effects of computer-based clinical decision support systems on clinician performance and patient outcome: a critical appraisal of research. *Archive of International Medicine*, 1994; 120:135–142

46. Evans RS, Classen DC, Pestotnik SL, Lundsgaarde HP, Burke JP, Improving empiric antibiotic selection using computer decision support. *Archive of International Medicine*, 1994; 154:878–884

47. Pestotnik SL, Classen DC, Evans RS, Burke JP, Implementing antibiotic practice guidelines through computer-assisted decision-support: clinical and financial outcomes. *Archive of International Medicine*, 1996; 124:884–890

48. Evans RS, Pestotnik SL, Classen DC, Clemmer TP, Weaver LK, Orme JF et al, A computer-assisted management program for antibiotics and other anti-infective agents. *New England Journal of Medicine*, 1998; 338:232–238

49. Shojania KG, Yokoe D, Platt R, Fiskio J, Ma'luf N, Bates DW, Reducing vancomycin use utilizing a computer guideline: results of a randomized controlled trial. *Journal of the American Medical Information Association*, 1998; 5:554–562

50. Bates DW, Leape LL, Cullen DJ, Laird N, Petersen LA, Teich JM et al, Effect of computerized physician order entry and a team intervention on prevention of serious medication errors. *Journal of the American Medical Association*, 1998; 280:1311–1316

51. Raschke RA, Gollihare B, Wunderlich TA, Guidry JR, Leibowitz AI, Peirce JC et al, A computer alert system to prevent injury from adverse drug events: development and evaluation in a community teaching hospital. *Journal of the American Medical Association*, 1998; 280:1317–1320

52. *The Way Forward for Hospital Pharmacy Services*, Department of Health, HC(88)54

53. Bond et al, Clinical pharmacy services and hospital mortality rates, *Pharmacotherapy*, 1999; 19: 556–564

54. Leape L et al, Pharmacist participation on physician rounds and adverse incidents in intensive care units, *Journal of the American Medical Association*, 1999; 282(3):267–270

55. Stevenson N, MSc thesis, Liverpool John Moores University, 1998

56. Stephens MJ et al, Managing medicines: the optimising drug value approach, *Hospital Pharmacist,* October 2000, Vol 7, 256–259

57. Fitzpatrick RW et al, A comprehensive system for managing medicines in secondary care, *Pharmaceutical Journal*, 2001; 266:585–588

58. Audit Commission, *A Prescription for Improvement – Towards more Rational Prescribing in General Practice*, Audit Commission/HMSO, 1994

59. Bowden JE, Reissuing patients' medicines – a step to seamless care. *Pharmaceutical Journal*, 1993, 251:356

60. Dobrzanski S, Reidy F, The pharmacist as a discharge medication planner in surgical patients. *Pharmaceutical Journal*, 1993; HS53–HS56

61. Campbell D et al, Waste not, want not, *Health Service Journal*, 24 August 2000, 31

62. HSC 2000/01:LAC (2001) *Intermediate Care*, Department of Health, January 2001

63. Lowe C et al, Effects of self-medication programme on knowledge of drugs and compliance with treatment in elderly patients, *British Medical Journal*, 1995; 310:1229–1231

64. Wood SI, Calvert RT, Acomb C, Kay EA, A self-medication scheme for elderly patients improves compliance with their medication regimens. *International Journal of Pharmacy Practice*, 1992; 1:240–1

65. Foster H, Mclean KA, Giles R, Franklin G, Auckland J, Neal KR et al, Self-medication does not improve drug compliance. Proceedings of Spring meeting of the British Geriatric Society, 1993. *Age and Ageing*, 1993; 22(suppl 3):23 [Abstract 65]

66. Rovelli M, Palmeri D, Vosser E, Bartus S, Hull D, Schweizer R, Non-compliance in organ transplant recipients. *Transplantation proceedings*, 1989; 21(no.1):833–834

67. Wright EC, How many aunts has Matilda? *Lancet*, 1993;342:909–13

68. Lowe C et al, Effects of self-medication programme on knowledge of drugs and compliance with treatment in elderly patients, *British Medical Journal*, 1995; 310:1229–1231

69. Wade B and Finlayson J, Drugs and the elderly, *Nursing Mirror*, 1983; 156, May:17–21

70. Bream S, Teaching the elderly about drugs. *Nursing Times*, 1985; 81 (29):32–34

71. Koltun A and Stone G, Past and current trends in patient noncompliance research, *The Journal of Compliance in Healthcare*, 1986; 1,(1), 22

72. Ausburn L, Patient compliance with medication regimes, *Advances in Behavioural Medicines*, 1981; Vol 1

73. NHS Management Executive, *Responsibility for Prescribing Between Hospitals and GPs*, EL(91)127, Department of Health, 1991

74. National hospital pharmacy vacancy survey 1999, conducted by the NHS Pharmacy Education and Development Committee

75. Royal College of Physicians, *Hospital Doctors Under Pressure: New Roles for the Healthcare Workforce*, 2000

76. Hughes DS et al, Collaborative medicines management: pharmacist prescribing, *Pharmaceutical Journal*; 263:170–172

77. Farrar KT, Stoddart M, Slee AL, Clinical pharmacy and re-active prescription review – time for a change? *Pharmaceutical Journal* 1998; 260:759–61

78. Cousins DH, Luscombe DK, *A New Model for Hospital Pharmacy Practice*, *Pharmaceutical Journal*, 1996; 256:347–51

79. *Health and Social Care Act*, The Stationery Office, 2001

80. Sayers D et al, Collaborative medicines management: pharmacist prescribing, *Pharmaceutical Journal*, 1999; 263:170–172

81. Slee AL, Farrar KT, *What are Normal Working Hours for Hospital Pharmacy?* *Pharmaceutical Journal*, 1998; 260:923–5

82. Department of Health, *Pharmacy Workforce and Training Report*, 1997

83. Department of Health, *Improved Working Lives Directive*, 2001

84. Audit Commission, *Finders, Keepers – The Management of Staff Turnover in NHS Trusts*, Audit Commission, 1997

85.   Bates DW et al, Using IT to reduce rates of medication errors in hospitals, *British Medical Journal*, 2000; 320:788–791

86.   Ford NG, Curtis C, Paul R, The Use of Electronic prescribing as part of a system to provide medicines management in secondary care. *British Journal of Hospital Care*, 2000; 17:26–28

87.   NHS Executive, *Information for health. An information strategy for the modern NHS 1998–2005*, September, 1998

88.   Abu Zayed L et al, Time spent on drug supply activities in UK hospitals, *American Journal of Health Systems Pharmacy*, 2000; 57:2006–7

89.   Department of Health, *Shifting the Balance of Power within the NHS*, 2001

Index References are to paragraph numbers, except in the case of boxes and case studies (page numbers)